Advanced Nursing Series
NURSING CARE OF ADULTS

Also available:
MODELS, THEORIES AND CONCEPTS
RESEARCH AND ITS APPLICATION
NURSING CARE OF CHILDREN

Advanced Nursing Series

NURSING CARE
OF ADULTS

Edited by

JAMES P. SMITH

OBE, BSc (Soc), MSc, DER, SRN, RNT
BTA Certificate, FRCN, FRSH

Editor of the *Journal of Advanced Nursing*
Visiting Professor of Nursing Studies
Bournemouth University

Blackwell
Science

This collection © 1996 by
Blackwell Science Ltd
Editorial Offices:
Osney Mead, Oxford OX2 0EL
25 John Street, London WC1N 2BL
23 Ainslie Place, Edinburgh EH3 6AJ
238 Main Street, Cambridge,
    Massachusetts 02142, USA
54 University Street, Carlton,
    Victoria 3053, Australia

Other Editorial Offices:
Arnette Blackwell SA
  1, rue de Lille, 75007 Paris
  France

Blackwell Wissenschafts-Verlag GmbH
  Kurfürstendamm 57
  10707 Berlin, Germany

  Feldgasse 13, A-1238 Wien
  Austria

First published 1996

Set by DP Photosetting, Aylesbury, Bucks
Printed and bound in Great Britain by
Hartnolls Ltd, Bodmin, Cornwall

DISTRIBUTORS
Marston Book Services Ltd
PO Box 87
Oxford OX2 0DT
(Orders: Tel: 01865 791155
        Fax: 01865 791927
        Telex: 837515)

North America
Blackwell Science, Inc.
238 Main Street
Cambridge, MA 02142
(Orders: Tel: 800 215-1000
         617 876 7000
    Fax: 617 492-5263)

Australia
Blackwell Science Pty Ltd
54 University Street
Carlton, Victoria 3053
(Orders: Tel: 03 347-0300
         Fax: 03 349 3016)

A catalogue record for this book is
available from the British Library

ISBN 0–632–03994–9

Library of Congress
Cataloging in Publication Data
Nursing care of adults/edited by James P. Smith.
        p.   cm.—(Advanced nursing series)
    Includes index.
    Contains updated papers originally published
in the Journal of advanced nursing.
    ISBN 0–632–03994–9
    1. Nursing.   I. Smith, James P., RNT.
II. Journal of advanced nursing.   III. Series.
    [DNLM: 1. Nursing Care—in adulthood—
collected works.   WY 100 N97478   1996]
RT63.N84   1996
610.73—dc20
DNLM/DLC
for Library of Congress   95-20836
                                            CIP

Contents

List of Contributors

Valerie Braithwaite, *PhD*
Senior Lecturer, Psychology Department, The Australian National University, Canberra, Australia.

Jane Christie, *RN, RCNT, DipN, BSc (Hons), PGDE, MSc*
Lecturer Practitioner – Trauma Services, Oxford Radcliffe Hospital, Oxford, England.

Carol Dealey, *BSc (Hons), SRN, RCNT*
Clinical Nurse Specialist in Tissue Viability, Community Hospitals Division, Southern Birmingham Community Health NHS Trust, Birmingham, England.

Jacquelyn H. Flaskerud, *RN, PhD*
Professor, School of Nursing, University of California, Los Angeles, California, USA.

Kathryn A. Getliffe, *PhD, MSc, BSc, RGN, DN Certificate*
Lecturer in Community Nursing, Department of Nursing and Midwifery, University of Surrey, Guildford, England.

Marilyn F. Jackson, *RN, BN, MEd*
Associate Professor, School of Nursing, University of Victoria, Victoria, British Columbia, Canada.

Patricia M. King, *RN, BN, MN*
Clinical Faculty, College of Nursing, University of Saskatchewan, Saskatoon, Canada.

Pekka Laippala, *PhD*
Associate Professor, Department of Public Health Biometry Unit, University of Tampere, Tampere, Finland.

Helen Leino-Kilpi, *PhD, RN*
Associate Professor, Department of Nursing, University of Turku, Turku, Finland.

Anne McGown, *MA*
Lecturer, Psychology Department, Faculty of Science, University of Canberra, Canberra, Australia.

Astrid Norberg, *RN, PhD*
Professor, Department of Advanced Nursing, Umeå University, Umeå, Sweden.

Linda A. Ross, *BA, RGN, PhD*
Research Fellow, Department of Management and Social Sciences, Queen Margaret College, Edinburgh, Scotland.

Evelyn Ruiz Calvillo, *RN, DNSc*
Professor, Department of Nursing, California State University, Los Angeles, California, USA.

James P. Smith, *OBE, BSc (Soc), MSc, DER, SRN, RNT, BTA Certificate, FRCN, FRSH*
Editor, *Journal of Advanced Nursing*, and Visiting Professor of Nursing Studies, Bournemouth University, England.

Anna Söderberg, *RNT*
Doctoral Student, Department of Advanced Nursing, Umeå University, Umeå, Sweden.

Tarja Suominen, *RN, PhD*
Assistant Professor, Department of Nursing, University of Turku, Turku, Finland.

Steven P. Wainwright, *MSc, BSc (Hons), PGCE, RGN*
Lecturer in Nursing Studies, Department of Nursing Studies, King's College, University of London, England.

Roger Watson, *BSc, PhD, RGN, CBiol, MIBiol*
Senior Lecturer, Department of Nursing Studies, The University of Edinburgh, Edinburgh, Scotland.

Introduction

JAMES P. SMITH

OBE, BSc(Soc), MSc, DER, SRN, RNT, BTA Certificate, FRCN, FRSH
Editor, *Journal of Advanced Nursing* and Visiting Professor of Nursing Studies,
Bournemouth University, England.

International problems and issues

The first two volumes in the Advanced Nursing Series were entitled *Models, Theories and Concepts* and *Research and its Application*. They were published in 1994.

This volume, *Nursing Care of Adults*, will complement those earlier publications. It consists of a collection of twelve scholarly papers which have been published in the *Journal of Advanced Nursing* in the past five years. The papers have been updated by their authors to form the twelve chapters of this volume.

The authors come from Australia, Canada, England, Finland, Scotland, Sweden and the USA. Their chapters are based on scholarly and research activities conducted in their own countries but, not surprisingly, the problems they focus on and the issues they raise are international problems and issues. Furthermore, as their reference lists illustrate, the chapters are supported by international literature sources.

The twelve chapters, written by nurses and others, will provide readers with sound knowledge bases for nursing practice. The delivery of knowledge-based nursing practice will undoubtedly enhance the delivery of quality nursing care to adults.

The chapters focus on a range of caring situations for men and women, young and older adults, who are suffering from physical and mental disorders requiring acute and long-term care in hospitals and in their own homes.

The art and science of nursing

When she was director of the nursing research unit at the University of Edinburgh, Scotland, Dr Lisbeth Hockey (1973) defined nursing science as 'a unique mix of other sciences with the uniqueness lying in the mix' and she argued that 'nursing is the art of applying nursing science'.

The contents of this book identify, illustrate and demonstrate the scientific elements of nursing science (or knowledge) and their application to the nursing care of a variety of patients in different health care settings.

The inevitability of the development of the science of nursing 'is written in nursing's long commitment to human health and welfare', as the American nursing scholar Dr M.E. Rogers (1970) has argued. She also points out that the rapid and unprecedented changes in health needs and health care have created a new urgency for the critical need for a body of scientific knowledge specific to nursing.

The contents of *Nursing Care of Adults* go some way to making a note-worthy contribution to nursing's body of knowledge that should help to promote excellent practice. The book should be of particular use – as a core textbook – for pre-registration nursing students, but it will also prove to be a valuable resource text for post-registration nursing students and practising nurses.

Health promotion

Health promotion is everybody's business and as Ms King from Canada says, in the opening chapter, health promotion is gaining recognition internationally as an important health care strategy. Indeed, health promotion should be integrated into every nursing curriculum.

Ms King discusses the concepts of health, wellness and disease prevention and she aims to develop an interest in health promotion from a nursing perspective. She points out that 'health is a relative, highly individualistic perception that is always evolving ... influenced by physiological, socio-cultural, spiritual and developmental domains and the interaction between each'. In the past, she says, nursing education programmes tended to be dominated by illness and pathology but now there is an increasing emphasis on wellness and the maintenance of health.

Ms King stresses that health promotion is a multidisciplinary activity which requires nurses to adopt a collaborative approach with other disciplines. That is a most important message for all nurses. Total care entails team care – provided by nurses, doctors, therapists, porters, chaplains, administrators and many informal carers (relatives, friends, neighbours and, increasingly, volunteers).

Ms King's message that a sound theoretical knowledge is essential for effective assessment, planning, implementation and evaluation of health promotion programmes is also a most important message for the whole of nursing practice.

Care at home

Most of every country's health care is provided in patients' homes where caregivers regularly give a great deal of care. In the UK, for example, there are probably five times as many home-based (unqualified) carers as there are registered nurses on the UK's register of nurses. The demands on caregivers at home increase each year as the population becomes more elderly and dependent. This demand is intensified by a greater emphasis, for a variety of political, social and economic reasons, on 'community care' programmes. Earlier discharge of patients from hospital and a greater use of day care services also adds to the demands made on the caregivers at home.

An example of home-based care is discussed in Chapter 2 by Dr Braithwaite and Ms McGown from Australia. They point out that home-based care for stroke patients has been recommended for a long time and increasingly stroke patients are being discharged from hospital as quickly as possible to continue their rehabilitation at home. Rehabilitation is important to assist the patients to independent living again. But, as the authors note, home care for stroke patients is not without problems. Those problems are common, in fact, when any patient is being cared for over a long period at home.

Responsibility for care is transferred to the family carer who often has no previous experience of caring. The carers have to make some adjustments. They have fears and anxieties and they suffer from a 'lack of information in a range of medical contexts'. All of this tends to militate against providing effective rehabilitation. The authors attempted to prevent information problems by providing information-giving seminars for the carers. Their study suggests that heightened emotionality of carers need not impair their capacity to care. The major challenge for nurses is to recognize the right time for providing information.

Nursing care problems

Chapters 3, 4 and 5 focus on three common problems facing nurses. Chapter 3, by Ms Dealey from England, considers the monitoring of the pressure sore problem. In Chapter 4 Dr Getliffe, also from England, discusses the implications of caring for patients with recurrent blockage of long-term urinary catheters. And Chapter 5 is devoted to a consideration of the feeding difficulties in patients with dementia, by Dr Watson from Scotland.

As Ms Dealey notes, pressure sores are a costly problem. Not only do pressure sores distress patients and increase morbidity but they are also a drain on health care resources. She indicates that the cost of treating one patient's deep sacral pressure sore equates with the cost of providing 17 hip or knee replacements. Yet, she points out, 95 per cent of pressure sores could be prevented. She has identified a number of factors related to tissue breakdown and makes a number of recommendations which should be noted.

Encrustation and subsequent blockage of indwelling urinary catheters is a common problem affecting up to 50% of long-term catheterized patients, Dr Getliffe points out. But long-term catheterization does offer a practical strategy for many people with urinary dysfunction where alternative non-invasive methods are inappropriate or ineffective. These patients form approximately 4% of the community nursing workload in the UK and up to 28% of patients in chronic care facilities. As a large number of these patients are elderly, the author points out that the percentages may well increase as the numbers of elderly people in the population increase.

Her study was conducted in an attempt to identify the 'blockers' early to assist in planning effective care strategies. She concludes that an individualized programme should be provided for all long-term catheterized patients; monitoring progress and care is fundamental to nursing practice, she says.

Not only will catheter care problems increase as the elderly people in the population increase, but so will the incidence of dementia, unfortunately. That has great implications for the work of nurses, as Dr Watson notes. He points out that elderly people suffering from dementia have nutritional problems and display changes in eating behaviour as the condition progresses. Ensuring that these patients not only have sufficient food but also are maintained in a healthy nutritional state is an important function of nurses. Research is still needed to identify appropriate nursing interventions. Dr Watson, in his study, used the Guttman scale to analyse the feeding difficulties. He suggests that the scoring system that was developed could well prove to be a useful tool for nurses.

Giving information and relieving pain

Chapters 6 and 7 deal with crucially important aspects of a nurse's responsibility to patients: the responsibilities for giving information to patients and ensuring that those in pain have that pain relieved.

Dr Suominen and colleagues from Finland draw attention to the importance of information for patients with breast cancer. But their contribution is also relevant to the care of all patients. They point out that cancer causes stress to patients and their families. Information is essential to enable them 'to devise realistic expectations'.

The study in Finland indicated that when breast cancer patients received appropriate information their recovery seemed to be better. But, if patients felt that they were not well informed before hospitalization, they were unable to ask the right kind of questions when they were inpatients. In fact, the patients' low levels of knowledge affected all aspects of their illness. 'Thus,' the authors conclude, 'by informing patients adequately, the hospital staff could compensate for knowledge gaps ... and support them on the road to recovery.'

Nowadays, there is sufficient knowledge about pain and the ways of relieving it for almost any patient to be maintained in a pain-free state. But, although methods of easing pain are relatively cheap, the journal *World Health* (1985) has pointed out that 'experience has shown that frequently physicians under-prescribe, and nurses under-dose, from apprehension that patients may become addicted to drugs'. It also claimed that 25% of all cancer patients still die with severe and unrelieved pain.

But, as Professor Calvillo and Professor Flaskerud from the USA point out in Chapter 7, there are important aspects of each country's 'culture' which impinge on individuals' responses to pain. As most countries now have populations consisting of a rich mix of many cultural and ethnic groups, all of whom are potential patients, it is important that nurses understand the ways that culture can affect the health status of individuals. For, as the authors point out, 'In each culture there is a way of life within which an individual may acquire attitudes, religious practices, language . . .' as well as responses to pain.

These views have been reiterated recently in the *Journal of Advanced Nursing* by Hussein Rassool (1995). He points out that the wide variation in life-style, health behaviour and language of ethno-cultural minorities affects perceptions and recognition of health problems and ill-health which have, he adds, been 'constructed within the paradigm of western medicine and health care system'.

Certainly, Professor Calvillo and Professor Flaskerud found that nurses judged pain differently based on the patient's ethnicity. The nurses also appeared to assign a greater amount of pain and more credibility to the expression of pain to those patients with 'more social value'. The authors conclude that nurses need to be more aware of how their own values and perceptions can affect how pain is treated.

Documentation

In Chapter 8, Ms Christie from England notes the importance of nursing documentation but concedes the difficulties. A particular difficulty is that nurses tend to devalue documentation in favour of 'patient care'. Yet there are legal implications if care is not adequately documented.

The problem seems to be greater in accident and emergency departments, so Ms Christie set about introducing and evaluating a nursing assessment tool to facilitate the documentation there. The quality of the documentation was measured by using the Phaneuf Audit Tool. The results of her study show that the introduction of the model achieved significant improvements in documentation and in the care patients received.

Organ transplantation

Organ transplantation has revolutionized the care available to many patients. But, as Mr Wainwright from England points out in Chapter 9, whilst liver transplantation is now the treatment of choice for patients with end-stage liver disease, it is also 'undoubtedly life changing, life threatening, and potentially life ending'. The first human liver transplant was performed in 1963 in the USA. The first one performed in the UK was in 1968. In 1990 about 3000 were performed worldwide – half in the USA.

Mr Wainwright's chapter clearly demonstrates that much knowledge can be gleaned from an exhaustive literature review. His contribution provides a wealth of information about how patients are evaluated for transplantation and how they recover and progress after the operation. He also notes the consequences for the patient's family. Unfortunately much of the literature has failed to capture the patient's own experience; that remains a challenge for future researchers.

Ethical problems

These days there is a growing recognition of the ethical problems associated with health care provision and treatment. The problems are many and varied. Solutions are not always easy but each individual health care practitioner has the personal responsibility for deciding whether or not their own actions or non-actions are correct human conduct. Students need time and opportunities to reflect on ethical problems. Teachers will provide an opportunity for this under their guidance. But if you are confronted with an ethical problem in your daily work, great relief and help will be found if the problem is shared. Friends, colleagues, teachers, chaplains and counsellors will all be willing to listen.

Ms Söderberg and Professor Norberg from Sweden, in Chapter 10, concede the difficulty of studying ethical reasoning in practice and share the outcome of a study of nurses and physicians working in intensive care units. The study demonstrated the effectiveness of using 'stories' about experience as a basis for discussion and analysis of ethically difficult caring situations. They note that the problems not only related to 'choice of action' (46%) but also to 'relationship problems' (54%). It is important to note that even though nurses and physicians shared certain perceptions, they did not share them with each other.

The authors conclude that narrating ethically difficult care episodes improves one's ability to perceive the complex patterns of care and is 'one way to make our personal values explicit and open to reflection and discussion'.

The spiritual dimension

Spiritual care is presented as part of the nurse's role by Dr Ross from
Scotland, in Chapter 11. She notes that a component of the spiritual
dimension is the need to find meaning, purpose and fulfilment (MPF) in life.
She argues that MPF is 'fundamental to the attainment of an optimum state
of health, wellbeing and quality of life'. Dr Ross also points out that the
International Council of Nurses and United Kingdom Central Council for
Nursing, Midwifery and Health Visiting have stressed, in their codes for
nurses, the importance of taking account of the 'spiritual beliefs' of patients
and clients. But she believes that an appropriate conceptual framework
should guide the nurse's practice.

Her study indicated that nurses seem able to identify spiritual needs and to
evaluate care given but they seem less willing to respond personally to the
spiritual needs of patients. Nonetheless, Dr Ross contends that the relief of
spiritual suffering would help achieve optimum health status.

Discharge planning

The final chapter in the book, by Associate Professor Jackson from Canada,
focuses on discharge planning for elderly patients. Adequate and advance
planning for all patients is essential in any health care programme in hospital.
'Discharge planning is a process and service where patient needs are identified and evaluated' to prepare the patient to move from one level of care to
another.

She endorses the view that planning for discharge must begin at least at the
time of admission to hospital. The plan must also be based on the reality of
the patient. It must also be flexible, especially in the case of elderly patients
where the 'need for flexibility and opportunity to revise a discharge plan is
paramount'.

The author also identifies a number of 'ethical questions' associated with
discharge planning. One ethical dilemma she notes relates to 'early' discharge
on the argument that it is cost-effective. But, she points out, the calculations
usually do not take into account the additional expenses of community-based
services and community nurses, nor do they include 'the cost to families who
are rapidly becoming unpaid givers of complex care'.

In spite of the growing amount of research on discharge planning, Ms
Jackson has identified several gaps in knowledge that need to be rectified.
These relate to standards, after-care, team effectiveness, and quality of life
issues – for patients and their families.

Conclusion

Those are the kind of challenges that will continue to confront nurses working in an ever changing, ever developing, cost-conscious health care system. For nurses have to learn to live with constant change and at the same time ensure that their role is cost-effective, adequate and appropriate for the care of patients and their families.

That requires them to be knowledgeable and inquisitive practitioners. It is also important that nurses recognize their role as an interdependent professional with others in the health care team, not only with other professional workers but also with the unpaid caregivers who give so much care to patients in their own homes.

References

Hockey, L. (1973) Nursing Research as a Basis for Nursing Science (unpublished paper). University of Edinburgh.

Rassool, G.H. (1995) The Health Status and Health Care of Ethno-Cultural Minorities in the United Kingdom: An Agenda for Action (guest editorial). *Journal of Advanced Nursing*, **21**, 199–221.

Rogers, M.E. (1970) *An Introduction to the Theoretical Basis of Nursing*. Davis, New York.

World Health (1985) Why not 'Freedom from cancer pain?' *World Health*, (June), 23–5.

Chapter 1
Health promotion: the emerging frontier in nursing

PATRICIA M. KING, *RN, BN, MN*

Clinical Faculty, College of Nursing, University of Saskatchewan, Saskatoon, Canada

Health promotion is gaining recognition as a health care strategy. The major premise of this chapter is that the nature of health promotion is emerging. Rising into view, health promotion offers many challenges and opportunities to all health care professionals. Many of the influences that health promotion will have on nursing have not yet been fully explored. What is health promotion? What concepts are inherent in health promotion? Are there models of health promotion that are specific to nursing? What will be nursing's role in health promotion? What changes are required by the nursing profession to enable nurses to emerge within this new frontier? These are central questions for nurses as health promotion professionals to ponder, and attempts are made in this chapter to answer these questions.

Emerging frontier

Health promotion, as an emerging frontier within the health care system, offers a challenge to the nursing profession. Nurses are summoned to alter their paradigm to 'a restructured health system and a shift from the predominant focus on illness and cure to an orientation toward wellness and care.' (Giordano & Igoe 1991). This change will take time and it will require an upstream futuristic view from the nursing profession.

The main objective of this chapter is to explore health promotion as an emerging paradigm in health care from a nursing perspective. Health, wellness and prevention will be discussed as they relate to health promotion. Clarification of health promotion as a concept is requisite to provide a sound theoretical knowledge base, and enables nurses to recognize health promotion as a phenomenon, to systematize observations and descriptions of health promotion, and to develop nursing behaviours inherent within the health promotion arena.

The intent of this chapter is to stimulate and further develop interest in health promotion from a nursing perspective. A brief review of key historical events will give credence for the existence of health promotion as a strategy to achieve health for all. Exploration of health promotion models exemplifies the concept as it relates to nursing. Nursing's role in health promotion is presented. Conclusions are made about the state of the art.

Historical evolution

> 'The concepts of health and health promotion have evolved from a historically rich background.' (Moore & Williamson 1984)

In 1974, *A New Perspective on the Health of Canadians* was released by Marc Lalonde, Canada's Minister of Health. The Lalonde document introduced the health field concept, which included the components of human biology, environment, lifestyle and health care organization. With each component equally weighted, the paper outlined the importance of the individual and society on determining health status (Lalonde 1974). As Raeburn (1992) clearly stated: 'The Lalonde report signalled the intention to move almost exclusive controlling power in the health field away from the medical profession and biomedicine to a wider field.' Although viewed as a 'signal' for the future, in that health was conceptually expanded, in reality the focus remained predominantly on the individual and biological determinants of health.

World Health Organization

In 1977, *Health for All By the Year 2000* was adopted by the World Health Organization (WHO 1978). The concept of primary health care was advocated by WHO at the Alma-Ata conference held in USSR in 1978. Since primary health care programmes provide promotive, preventive, curative and rehabilitative services, primary health care has been viewed as an important delivery strategy for achieving 'health for all' (WHO 1978; Little 1992). Equity in distribution and accessibility of all programmes were identified as key concepts in primary health care. The declaration was made 'against a background of evidence that health care resources are too concentrated in centralized, professionally dominated, high technological institutions . . . at the expense of access . . . at the local, community level' (Green & Raeburn 1990).

Canadian document

In 1986, the Canadian document entitled *Achieving Health For All: A Framework for Health Promotion* was released by Jake Epp, the Minister of

National Health & Welfare. This framework identified health promotion as a multifaceted intervention designed to respond to the national health challenges of reducing inequities, increasing prevention and enhancing coping. Epp offered broad-based strategies and mechanisms that, if achieved by Canadians, could improve health and quality of life. Health promotion was seen as an approach to health care (Epp 1986). Epp clearly introduced the idea that achieving healthful states was both a personal and societal responsibility. Epp's framework was an attempt to squash the 'victim blaming' which resulted from the heavy focus on individual behaviour following Lalonde's health field concept. In contrast, Epp clearly addressed the fact that some people have unequal opportunities for achieving healthful states and that health is often related to factors beyond the individual's control. Epp's framework, which was presented later in 1986 at the International Health Promotion Conference in Ottawa, became known as the 'Ottawa Charter'. The framework has since been viewed as a working document for action to achieve 'health for all' by the year 2000 and beyond (International Conference on Health Promotion 1986). The framework will be explored in greater detail later.

Societal trends

Although these papers were formulated to meet political and social agendas of the day, societal trends had important influences. Advances in medical science contributed to the changing nature of diseases: infectious diseases were decreasing while chronic illness was on the rise. To accept a broader conceptualization of health, people began to look critically at their lifestyles and the influence of their behaviours on health. Capitalizing on this, the media focused on youth, fitness and 'wise' lifestyle choices. Health and wellness were considered to be in vogue.

> 'The era of health promotion has been ushered in as a social movement, and much of its impetus has arisen from persons and institutions outside the medical mainstream.' (Taylor *et al.* (1982)

The change in focus, from illness to wellness, has been described as a 'medical nemesis' by Illich (1976).

As well as being a health-care strategy, health promotion has gained momentum as a social movement with political overtones. Understanding the concepts inherent within health promotion is imperative.

Concept clarification

Health

> 'Health ... is a crucial, though incredibly complicated, concept in our understanding of "health promotion".' (de Leeuw 1989)

Review of the literature reveals some major trends in the conceptual development of health. Health has evolved on four dimensions: (a) absolute versus relative notion of health; (b) subjective versus objective; (c) individual versus societal responsibility; and (d) unidimensional versus holistic.

An absolute notion of health can be seen as dichotomous: either one is healthy or ill. In 1978, WHO defined health as a 'state of complete physical, mental and social wellbeing'. This 'complete', absolute state has been criticized as somewhat unachievable, irrelevant and idealistic (O'Grady 1985; Maglacas 1988; de Leeuw 1989). The traditional orientation toward illness has reinforced the health-illness dichotomy as 'both health care providers and receivers have traditionally viewed health from an illness perspective' (Tatro & Gleit 1983). The biomedical model has viewed health from a reductionistic, dichotomous perspective where mind and body are separate (Shaver 1985).

Over time, health evolved within the sociopolitical context and was viewed relatively, as opposed to a dual state of health or illness. Health moved from being perceived as an absolute, negative concept to a positive, relative one involving a balance between body and mind. Psychology contributed to the concept of health, as it was viewed dynamically with the contention that health is everchanging and influenced by individual factors such as adaptive potential and perceptual capability, stressors and the environment. Dunn (1959) held a dynamic view and defined health as an integrated method of human functioning that maximized the individual's potential (Eberst 1984). Other relative notions were the optimum potentialization views of Nightingale (1938) and Maslow (1962) and the adaptation view of Dubos (1965). Each of these views clearly recognized the individual's subjective contribution as well as the objective, environmental influences on health. The multidimensionality of health was recognized.

An integrated biopsychosocial view of health emerged. Shaver (1985) noted that this view of health was individualistic yet comprehensive, since the influence of biology, psychology and sociology were recognized. This view of health suggested that:

> 'many of the factors that affect the health of individuals arise from sectors traditionally considered outside the field of health concerns. If these factors are not incorporated into new approaches to health, the potential for improvement of the health of individuals will be limited.' (Doucette 1989)

With the societal and environmental influences on health realized, it became necessary to look beyond the signs and symptoms of diseases to the root of causes. Health was viewed more holistically.

Lalonde (1974) formulated a functionalist view of health. Within this view the components of human behaviour, environment, lifestyle and health care organization presented a new and comprehensive perspective on health. The 'fragments are brought together into a unified whole which permits everyone to see the importance of all factors' (Lalonde 1974). One of the unique aspects of Lalonde's health field concept was the recognition of lifestyle as a powerful determinant of health. Inherently, the power base was shifted to a wider base of control: the people themselves. Interestingly, Chalmers & Farrell (1983) noted that perception of control is an important determinant of health outcomes and will influence health promotion activities. Within Lalonde's view, health was clearly recognized to be holistic yet subjective, notwithstanding the combined responsibility of the individual as well as the environment.

WHO's (1986) current definition of health has moved beyond the biological causes, and views health more holistically with a relative stance. Health is:

> 'the extent to which an individual or group is able, on the one hand, to realize aspirations and satisfy needs; and, on the other hand, to change or cope with the environment … a resource for everyday life, not the objective of living … a positive concept emphasizing social and personal resources, as well as physical capacities.'

In the context of health promotion, health has been considered 'less as an abstract state and more in terms of the ability to achieve one's potential and to respond positively to the challenges of the environment' (de Leeuw 1989).

In summary, health is a relative, highly individualistic perception that is always evolving. From a holistic perspective, health is influenced by physiological, psychological, sociocultural, spiritual and developmental domains and the interaction between each. Health, subjectively and objectively, is viewed as the ability to balance the forces of each domain within the environmental context, and the outcome of balancing may be truly perceived only by the individual experiencing it.

Wellness

Wellness is another important concept related to health and health promotion. Although, wellness and health have often been equated as similar, health and health care which have an illness orientation have concentrated on negatives. In contrast 'wellness is from a very different focus: positive engagement in behaviors to enhance an even higher feeling of wellness, i.e.

accentuating the positive instead of merely eliminating the negative.' (Tatro & Gleit 1983).

Dunn (1973) has been regarded by some to be the father of the wellness movement (Moore & Williamson 1984). Lane (1992) further recognized Dunn's contribution, as wellness was seen as 'an integrated method of functioning, oriented toward maximizing the potential of which an individual is capable' through balanced and purposeful direction within their environment. Uniqueness rests in the person's potential to achieve a state of wellness. In achieving a wellness state, Dunn emphasized the important determinants of personality, motivation, environment, dynamics and change (Dunn 1973). Therefore, wellness is a qualitative concept, closely related to quality of life:

> 'Wellness refers to our physical, mental and spiritual well-being. It means getting healthy and staying healthy. Wellness means improving our quality of life.' (Simard 1992b)

Somewhat intangible for professionals and self-defined by individuals, a wellness approach is crucial to understanding and implementing health promotion. As Brubaker (1983) outlined, wellness care encompasses health promotion, health maintenance and disease prevention.

Prevention

Primary, secondary and tertiary prevention, as proposed by Leavell & Clarke in 1965, have an illness orientation; according to Webster's Dictionary (1992), to prevent means 'to stop or intercept'. The three levels of prevention were derived from an epidemiological perspective that is rooted in the biomedical model. Disease prevention tends to view health absolutely and efforts are aimed at a specific risk group susceptible to a certain disease pathology. Epidemiological methods are used to study and evaluate prevention strategies.

Primary prevention takes place before a disease process starts, with the goal being the prevention of the occurrence of the disease. Secondary prevention begins after a disease is present and the goal is to lessen complications and disability. Early diagnosis and prompt treatment are the major foci. With tertiary prevention or rehabilitation, which begins when the disease process has stabilized, the goal is to restore the highest level of functioning possible (Leavell & Clarke 1965).

Primary prevention has ties within the realm of health promotion, since both involve protection from disease and activities geared toward increasing the general level of health and wellbeing of an individual, family or community (Leavell & Clarke 1965). The target population for primary prevention is viewed as healthy. Shamansky & Clausen (1980) identified primary prevention as including 'generalized health promotion as well as specific protection against disease'. This conceptual overlapping and the existing semantic struggle results in ambiguity and ultimately hinders the understanding of the relationship between the two concepts. Obviously, health professionals must view health promotion and disease prevention as complementary concepts that are not mutually exclusive.

'Any program of health promotion or disease prevention may bear some components of the other' (Stachtchenko & Jenicek 1990).

Health promotion

Health promotion is difficult to define. Nevertheless, nurses require a solid theoretical foundation of this concept if full understanding and involvement are to be achieved. The term health promotion has often been used interchangeably with disease prevention, health maintenance and health education. This contributes to conceptual ambiguity. Brubaker (1983) argued that 'the term health promotion is not synonymous with disease prevention, health maintenance, primary prevention or health education. It is a term that refers to a specific area of health care.' Health promotion involves all of these activities.

As a separate entity within health care, health promotion is 'directed toward growth and improvement in wellness' (Brubaker (1983). Health promotion involves movement toward a positive state of health and wellbeing. 'Health promotion seems to have become an all inclusive umbrella term under which any health service may find coverage' (Duncan & Gold 1986).

While it has been noted that health promotion and disease prevention are complementary, it is important to note that the goal of health promotion has a broader focus. Health-promoting activities strive to increase one's state of health, whereas disease prevention strives to maintain the *status quo*. Methodological approaches to study and evaluate health promotion are less developed than those for disease prevention. While disease prevention research focuses on specific disease processes, health promotion research addresses general health. Clarke (1992) revealed that health promotion research is based on positivism. Positivism is 'rooted in a belief that it is possible to observe, describe, quantify and explain the social world as if it were objectively real, external and immoveable' (Clarke 1992).

Health promotion is concerned with people and their wellbeing from their perspective (Raeburn 1992). In health promotion, health is viewed as a positive construct and involves people in a participatory capacity. As participants, people are to be given as much control as possible (or desirable) to achieve health or a higher state of wellness. Health promotion is 'grounded in philosophies of individual and community control of health' (Townsend 1992). The quest for health and wellness, within the health promotion arena, becomes a responsibility of the collective as well as the individual. Both societal and individual perceptions of health and wellness and perceived health status must be assessed.

Social expectation

Behavioural components play an important role in health promotion, but social, economic and ecological contexts also influence the process. Guidotti (1989) outlined the process of 'health promotion as a powerful [one] because it places a positive emphasis on enhanced wellbeing as a social expectation'. Health promotion can be viewed as a moral responsibility. At the environmental level health promotion is the 'development of an environment that is conducive to overall wellness' (Duffy 1988). Here, change in the social structure or environment is implied to be an important goal of health promotion activities.

Although personal control and choice are implicit within health promotion, the focus has been extended to include a global perspective. Health promotion is not apolitical, rather it is an explicitly, politically orientated activity. Certainly, this should not be masqueraded, leaving the consumer (or provider) wondering about hidden agendas. Governments decide agendas and simply 'it is the authorities that set the priorities' (Parish *et al.* 1991). Government agencies tend to portray a utilitarian attitude to consumers of health, citing the most good for the greatest number as impetus for changes that occur in health care. Nevertheless, the fully informed health care consumer will probably perceive more control over health and participate in a greater capacity. While information may not always lead to participation, it is a requisite for perceived control and participation. Further, health consumers and health providers may be increasingly expected to become political and social activists in order to gain control and influence the factors that affect people's health. To reiterate, the responsibility for health is both societal and individual.

Health promotion is multisectoral, requiring a broad and holistic conceptualization of health and health care by consumers and providers. The whole is more than the sum of the parts. 'An expanded view of health considers factors such as housing, employment, education and the environment.' (Simard 1992b). Further, this 'broader view of health also includes empowered health consumers and health professionals, and a new generation of health services' (Simard 1992a). Within this expanded paradigm, the biomedical model of health care is obsolete. Crippling a holistic approach, the medical model can be viewed as iatrogenic. For this reason, there is a distinct need to re-orientate the delivery of health care beyond the curative focus that the medical model dictates.

Defining health promotion

There have been many definitions of health promotion that have emerged in the literature over the past number of years. Exploration of these will clarify some of the characteristics that health promotion activities claim to possess. WHO (1986) defined health promotion as 'the process of enabling people to increase control over the determinants of health and thereby improve their health.' Health promotion, then, involves enabling and empowering people to take control over their health. Indeed, the goal of health promotion is increased wellbeing.

Another definition of health promotion is 'the organized application of educational, social and environmental resources enabling individuals to adopt and maintain behaviours that reduce risk of disease and enhance wellness.' (Petosa 1986). Therefore, health promotion is organized and multidimensional. Health promotion involves many activities, including health education, maintenance and protection, community and environmental development, research and healthy public policy. Health promotion can be viewed as a means to an end: a distinct entity in health care to achieve 'health for all'.

Health promotion models

Achieving health for all

In the paper entitled *Achieving Health For All: A Framework for Health Promotion*, health promotion was seen as an approach to complement the existent health care system (Epp 1986). The framework outlined three health challenges for Canadians: reducing inequities, increasing prevention and enhancing coping. These challenges were offered as a means for Canadians to achieve health and improve their quality of life. To meet these challenges, Epp identified health promotion strategies.

Health promotion strategies involved activities such as self-care, mutual aid and healthy environments. To encourage people to care for themselves and to come together for mutual aid to change their environments, Epp suggested fostering public participation, strengthening community health services and co-ordinating public policies (Epp 1986).

Epp's framework, which has a community and global orientation, respects the federal and provincial responsibilities in health. The framework links together the concepts of health promotion, healthy policy and healthy environments to achieve health for all.

Epp's framework focuses on environmental influences as a central concern in achieving healthful states. In this framework, health challenges are not posed in terms of individual responsibilities; rather, they reflect broader societal responsibilities. Nevertheless, there is a need for more specific information on how to implement the framework in practice. There is a need for further quantitative research on the framework.

'The framework is not formal policy and there have been no additional resources to help move health promotion from the periphery of the health field to a central position as a cornerstone of policy.' (Pinder 1988)

A Saskatchewan Vision For Health

In 1992, the Saskatchewan Minister of Health, Louise Simard, released a position paper entitled *A Saskatchewan Vision For Health: A Framework for Change*. The 'vision' has been proposed as a way to restructure and reorganize health care in Saskatchewan. Simard incorporates a definition of health that 'includes an individual's physical, mental, social, cultural, economic, and spiritual wellbeing' (Simard 1992a).

The goals of the *Saskatchewan Vision For Health* include comprehensiveness, universality, portability, accessibility, and public administration of health care. The vision cited the 'wellness approach' to enhance the health of the province's people and achieve health for all. 'Flexibility, support for local initiatives, respect for diversity, and responsiveness to identified health needs guide the reform process' (Simard 1992b). Simard's vision, as a provincial operationalization of Epp's framework, has recognized the societal and community roles without ignoring or neglecting the importance of individual commitment and participation. Simard (1992a) has identified the activities of education, training, research, and community development as inherent within health promotion.

The political agenda – the reduction of health care costs – is outlined by Simard (1992a,b) who cited the escalating costs of health care as challenging economic realities and the driving force for change. As DeFriese (1986) noted though, health promotion programmes are often 'sold' as cost reduction measures. Whether or not this 'vision' is politically and economically feasible has yet to be determined. To this point, no quantitative research findings could be found to support the notion that health promotion is indeed cost-effective. Nevertheless, health reform and renewal processes are occurring at a rapid pace throughout Canada.

Health promotion, through regionalization, is the key principle guiding the changes in the way health care is managed and delivered. Jackson (1995) noted that in one year, 1992 to 1993, Saskatchewan moved from 400 assorted boards to 30 district health boards. The Saskatchewan district health planning committees and boards have been formulated so that health services can be developed, managed and utilized in a more consistent and coordinated manner. The goals to be achieved through the consolidation of services include:

(1) Increased community based services thereby fostering empowerment of the consumer through grass roots involvement.
(2) Prevention of the duplication of services.
(3) Cost reduction.

Through these goals, the 'vision' is becoming a reality.

Health promotion model

Nola Pender developed a health promotion model in 1982 and made revisions in 1987 (Pender 1987). The model is one of the predominant models of health promotion in nursing. The model was proposed as an explanation of why individuals engage in health behaviour. Pender viewed cognitive–perceptual factors, modifying factors and other variables as determinants of behaviour affecting the likelihood of action:

> 'Cognitive–perceptual factors are identified in the model as the primary motivational mechanisms for acquisition and maintenance of health promoting behaviours.' (Pender 1987)

Modifying factors exert their influence through cognitive–perceptual mechanisms that directly affect behaviour. Pender's model viewed health promotion as an approach behaviour that 'consists of activities directed toward increasing the level of well being and actualizing the health potential of individuals, families, communities, and society' (Pender 1987).

While the health promotion model provides an organizing framework for theory development and research in health promotion behaviour, it is incongruent with Epp's framework for health promotion. Unlike Epp, who viewed the environment as a crucial concern, Pender viewed environment, situational and interpersonal factors as modifiers of the central cognitive–perceptual factors. Pender viewed the environment as it relates to behaviour rather than how it relates to health.

Unlike Epp, Pender gave little recognition to the impact that the socio-political context has on the individual. Rather, Pender focused on individuals, their perception of control, their definition of health, and their decision-making capacity. Pender (1987) admitted that the extent to which the model can explain lifestyle patterning or specific behaviours remains to be seen. The model neglected to address the behaviour of families and communities, which are important influences on individual behaviour. Pender's model is further limited as the existence or complexity of inter-relationships among the factors is not acknowledged. For example, how do interpersonal influences relate to one's definition of health? Is one's age reflected in one's definition of health? The model also does not specifically address motivating factors. Is motivation intrinsic? Hilton (1986) felt that further clarification was needed in the area of self-esteem and questioned 'do attitudes precede behavioural change, or vice versa, or do they alternate?'

There is a need for health promotion models to move beyond assessment of health and health programmes; there is a need to implement these pro-grammes and movement must be made towards such implementation. Fur-ther, there is a need to develop a dynamic balance between the individual and global foci. The individual and global environmental context should be considered to be of equal account (Green & Raeburn 1990). As de Leeuw (1989) noted, there is an inextricable link between persons and their envir-onment; this link is of central importance to the concept of health promotion. Within the collaborative frontier of health promotion, there is a need for all disciplines involved to work together to develop a multidisciplinary health promotion model that can be shared but is specific enough to delineate the amenable interventions for each involved discipline.

Nursing's role in health promotion

In keeping with the emerging frontier of health promotion 'health can no longer be seen by practising nurses as a process to be dealt with only when it has broken down' (O'Grady 1985). Nursing in the emerging frontier of health promotion requires a broader view:

> 'The pressure is on for a shift by nurses from their traditional roles to the assumption of greater responsibility in a much wider arena of action focusing on healthy people and healthy environments.' (Doucette (1989)

Simard (1992b) also addressed the expansion of nursing roles and has stated, 'nurses will increasingly be the primary health team members in many communities ... assuming other expanded roles where required'. Saskatch-ewan nurses are left with many questions: What kind of role changes is Simard advocating for nurses? Will nursing roles be more dilute or more specialized? How will nurses be trained to 'assume' expanded roles? How will these changes evolve? Is Simard advocating the need for nurse practitioners? How will the government compensate nurses for expansion in roles? The frontier of health promotion is uncertain yet exciting and:

> ... guides the nurse and client away from a definition of health as the absence of disease and towards a concern for generalized wellbeing ... enhancement of wellbeing in the presence of absence of disease becomes a legitimate arena for nursing practice, research, and education (Duffy 1988)

In these arenas – practice, research and education – there are specific roles and opportunities for nurses as health promotion professionals. In all arenas nurses are challenged to emerge or rise above the traditional theoretical frame of reference of nursing.

Practice

Nurses in practice must be 'committed to community involvement and development' (Doucette 1989). Nurses are invited to act as role models, educators, advocators, problem solvers and facilitators. Maglacas (1988) stressed that nurses should run healthy health services, not illness services. To do this:

> 'nurses will need to develop new skills ... in enabling and empowering people for self care, self help, and environmental improvement and in promoting positive health behaviour and appropriate coping abilities of people to maintain health.' (Maglacas 1988)

While empowering these people nurses must respect the individuality of each person.

> 'People learn and become involved in a healthy lifestyle when they are ready, for their own reasons, and progress at their own pace.' (Green 1985)

Nurses must realize that health promotion is not the sole responsibility of nursing:

> 'Empowering communities to take control of their health means giving them control over programmes' (Labonte 1987).

Pender's (1987) model of health promotion for nursing is one that stresses the individual's control over 'complexity, variation, and meaningfulness of stimuli within their environment.' Nurses are in a prime position, though, to explore these factors with individuals and communities.

Other skills for practising nurses will include information dissemination and mediation for healthy public policy formation (Spellbring 1991). As Lefebrve (1991) warned:

> 'Health educator, social marketer, and politician, all in equal parts, will be the characteristics of the community health promotion professional who is effective and successful in the 1990s.'

Butterfield (1990) further stated that 'involvement in social reform is considered to be within the realm of nursing practice'. As social activists, nurses must lobby and participate in role clarification within the realm of health promotion practice.

'To be successful, nurses need to understand better the agendas and priorities of key decision makers and others who influence public policy.' (Maglacas 1988)

Additionally, 'political activism must be seen as a mode of nursing practice' (Williams 1989). Nurses in their role as community health promotion professionals will be involved in needs assessment, organizing and integrating existing services, marketing programmes, and choosing appropriate locations (Igoe & Giordano 1992).

Education

In education, strategies to teach health promotion as a nursing role need to be formulated. The theory of health promotion cannot be dichotomized from the practice of health promotion. Practical skills to fulfil the health promotion role and all of its components, such as counselling, educating and managing, need to be taught from a health promotion perspective. Experts contend that a course on health promotion for all students of nursing would be desirable (Pender *et al.* 1992). Parish *et al.* (1991) noted that nurses must adopt and exercise healthy lifestyles to promote their function as exemplars so as to avoid loss of credibility as health educators. Parish *et al.* (1991) felt that 'particular attention should be given to their exemplar role during basic training'. Nursing education must change with the times. Basic nursing education needs to stress the importance of promotive, preventive, curative, rehabilitative and managerial services (Doucette 1989). Nurses who graduate with the knowledge that they have 'unique skills and a unique position to help themselves and others attain and maintain the balance and perspective associated with a state of wellness' (Fritz 1984) will be in a stronger position to make significant contributions to health promotion initiatives.

Research

Nurses could play a crucial role in studying the concepts and behaviours inherent in health promotion to build on the existent theoretical knowledge base. Nurse researchers must encourage non-researchers to become involved to foster community participation (Eakin & Maclean 1992). Health promotion is people-orientated and it is incumbent upon nurse researchers to strive to maintain this orientation. Harris (1992) felt that qualitative research paradigms satisfied the naturalistic context of health promotion activities. More of such research is needed to build the theoretical knowledge base of health promotion. Nurses, with 'hands on' interactions with individuals, families and communities are in a unique position to carry out such research.

'Through research focused on health and health promotion, nurses can create an improvement in the wellbeing of individuals, families and communities.' (Duffy 1988)

Conclusion: the state of the art

Health promotion is a complex concept. Clearly, it:

'is more than the adoption of positive health habits or the avoidance of negative health behaviours. Health promotion involves a complicated web of knowledge, attitudes, and behaviour related to health (Kulbok & Baldwin 1992)

Review of this web leads to some important conclusions about health promotion.

Knowledge

Health promotion is emerging as a politically orientated health care strategy. As such, opportunities for research abound. Nursing research that focuses on the complex interrelationships among relevant concepts such as health, wellness, disease prevention, health behaviour, health maintenance, health protection, lifestyle, self-care, empowerment and control will enhance the theoretical knowledge on health promotion as a nursing phenomenon.

Attitudes

The nursing profession has historically been rooted in the provision of disease-oriented care within individual nurse–client relationships under the dictatorship of the biomedical model. Traditionally, nursing theory has as its foundation the nurse–client relationship, with specific emphasis placed on the client as an individual. Nursing in the 1990s, though, holds a broader conceptualization of the client and, increasingly, the client is recognized as individual, group, family or community. Health, too, has evolved into a broader conceptualization. Health is viewed as a relative, subjective, holistic concept for which the individual and society have responsibility. With these and other evolving concepts, nursing is realizing the truly infinite scope of the nursing profession within health promotion.

Behaviour

Health promotion is multidisciplinary and nurses will be required to adopt a collaborative approach with other disciplines. Before this can be accomplished, nursing must first embrace and then further develop the concepts of health, wellness and client from a nursing perspective. When the developed concepts are accepted, in theory and in practice, nursing will more fully grasp the collaborative nature that health promotion requires. As Butterfield (1990) contended, nursing has to reconcile the difference between popula-tion-centred practice and nursing theories that primarily define nursing in terms of individually focused care. When this reconciliation is made, nurses will be recognized for the invaluable contributions made on multidisciplinary teams. All involved disciplines will need to work together with clients to develop and formulate common models for health promotion practice.

When nursing is ready to participate collaboratively with other disciplines (and these disciplines are ready for nursing), nursing behaviours will need to be clearly developed. Indeed, nurses are capable of fulfilling many roles in the health promotion arena. The emerging scope of the role of nursing offers both uncertainty and excitement. Changes are required and change is rarely easy. Nurses will be required to perfect their enabling, empowering promo-tive skills. A sound theoretical base of knowledge will be essential as nurses link theory to the practice endeavours of assessment, planning, and imple-mentation and evaluation.

Nurses must examine what health promotion has to offer as well as what nursing can offer health promotion. Role clarification and specification are necessary if nurses are to embark upon this emerging frontier.

Acknowledgements

The author would like to acknowledge Wilda Watts and Dr. Karen Semchuk.

References

Brubaker, B.H. (1983) Health promotion: a linguistic analysis. *Advances in Nursing Science*, **5**(3), 1–14.

Butterfield, P.G. (1990) Thinking upstream: nurturing a conceptual understanding of the societal context of health behaviour. *Advances in Nursing Science*, **12**(2), 1–8.

Chalmers, K. & Farrell, P. (1983) Nursing interventions for health promotion. |*Nurse Practi-tioner*, **8**(10), 62.

Clarke, J.N. (1992) Feminist methods in health promotion research. *Canadian Journal of Public Health*, **83**(Suppl. 1), 54–7.

DeFriese, G.H. (1986) Cost-effectiveness as a basis for assessing the policy significance of health promotion. In *Advances in Health Education and Promotion*. (Ed. W.B. Wold), pp. 7–21. JAI Press, Connecticut.

Doucette, S. (1989) The changing role of nurses: the perspective of the medical services branch. *Canadian Journal of Public Health*, **80**(2), 92–4.

Dubos, R. (1965) *Man Adapting*. Yale University Press, Connecticut.

Duffy, M.E. (1988) Health promotion in the family: current findings and directives for nursing research. *Journal of Advanced Nursing*, **13**(1), 109–17.

Duncan, D.F. & Gold, R.S. (1986) Reflections: health promotion – What is it? *Health Values*, **10**(3), 47–8.

Dunn, H.L. (1959) High-level wellness in man and society. *American Journal of Public Health*, **49**, 786.

Dunn, H.L. (1973) *High Level Wellness.* Beatty, Virginia.

Eakin, J.M. & Maclean, H.M. (1992) A critical perspective on research and knowledge development in health promotion. *Canadian Journal of Public Health*, **83**(suppl. 1), 572–6.

Eberst, R.M. (1984) Defining health: a multidimensional model. *Journal of School Health*, **54**(3), 99–104.

Epp, J. (1986) Achieving health for all: a framework for health promotion. *Canadian Journal of Public Health*, **77**(6), 393–430.

Fritz, W.S. (1984) Maintaining wellness. *Nursing Clinics of North America*, **19**, 263–9.

Giordano, B.P. & Igoe, J.B., (1991) Health promotion: the new frontier. *Pediatric Nursing*, **17**, 490–92.

Green, K. (1985) Health promotion: its terminology, concepts and modes of practice. *Health Values*, **9**(3), 8–14.

Green, L.W. & Raeburn, J. (1990) Contemporary developments in health promotion. In *Health Promotion at the Community Level* (Ed. N. Bracht), pp. 29–44. Sage, Newbury Park, California.

Guidotti, T.L. (1989) Health promotion in perspective. *Canadian Journal of Public Health*, **80**, 400–405.

Harris, E.M. (1992) Assessing community development research methodologies. *Canadian Journal of Public Health*, **83**(suppl. 1), 62–6.

Hilton, A. (1986) Analysis of Pender's health-promotion behaviour model. *Nursing Papers*, **18**(1), 57–66.

Igoe, J.B. & Giordano, B.P. (1992) Health promotion and disease prevention: secrets of success. *Pediatric Nursing*, **18**(1), 61–2.

Illich, I. (1976) *Limits to Medicine–Medical Nemesis: The Expropriation of Health.* Penguin, New York.

International Conference on Health Promotion (1986) *Ottawa Charter.* International Conference on Health Promotion, Ottawa, Ontario, Canada.

Jackson, R.A. (1995). The heartbeat of reform. *The Canadian Nurse*, **91**(3), 23–32.

Kulbok, P.A. & Baldwin, J.H. (1992) From preventive health behaviour to health promotion: Advancing a positive construct of health. *Advances in Nursing Science*, **14**(4), 50–64.

Labonte, R. (1987) Community health promotion strategies. *Health Promotion*, **26**, 5–9, 32.

Lalonde, M. (1974) *A New Perspective on the Health of Canadians.* Information Canada, Ottawa.

Lane, B. (1992) Health and wellness in the city. In *Perspectives on Urban Health* (Ed. B. Mathur), pp. 5–12. University of Winnipeg, Winnipeg.

Leavell, H.R. & Clarke, E.G. (1965) *Preventative Medicine for the Doctor in His Community.* Mcgraw-Hill, New York.

de Leeuw, E. (1989) Concepts in health promotion: the notion of relativism. *Social Science and Medicine*, **29**, 1281–8.

Lefebrve, R.C. (1991) Promoting health promoters: professional development in health promotion. *Health Promotion International*, **6**(1), 1–2.

Little, C. (1992) Health for all by the year 2000: Where is it now? *Nursing and Health Care*, **13**, 198–201.

Maglacas, A.M. (1988) Health for all: nursing's role. *Nursing Outlook*, **36**(2), 66–71.

Maslow, A.H. (1962) *Toward a Psychology of Being.* D. Van Nostrand, Princeton, New Jersey.

Moore, P.V. & Williamson, G.C. (1984) Health promotion: evolution of a concept. *Nursing Clinics of North America*, **19**, 195–206.

Nightingale, F. (1938) *Notes on Nursing: What it is and what it is not.* Appleton, New York.

O'Grady, T.P. (1985) Health versus illness: nurses can chart a course for the future. *Nursing and Health Care*, **6**, 318–21.

Parish, R., Powell, C. & Wilkes, E. (1991) Health promotion in nursing practice. *Nursing Standard*, **5**(23), 37–40.

Pender, N.J. (1987) *Health Promotion in Nursing Practice*, 2nd edn. Appleton & Lange, Norwalk, Connecticut.

Pender, N.J. Barauskas, V.H., Hayman, L., Rice, V.H. & Anderson, E.T. (1992) Health promotion and disease prevention: toward excellence in nursing practice and education. *Nursing Outlook*, **40**, 106–12.

Petosa, R. (1986) Emerging trends in adolescent health promotion. *Health Values*, **10**(3), 22–8.

Pinder, L. (1988) From a new perspective to the framework: a case study on the development of health promotion in Canada. *Health Promotion*, **3**, 205–12.

Raeburn, J. (1992) Health promotion research with heart: keeping a people perspective. *Canadian Journal of Public Health*, **83**(suppl. 1), 20–24.

Shamansky, S.L. & Clausen, C.L. (1980) Levels of prevention: examination of a concept. *Nursing Outlook*, **28**, 104–108.

Shaver, J.F. (1985) A biopsychosocial view of human health. *Nursing Outlook*, **33**, 186–91.

Simard, L. (1992a) *A Saskatchewan Vision for Health: Challenges and Opportunities*. Saskatchewan Health, Regina.

Simard, L. (1992b) *A Saskatchewan Vision for Health: A Framework for Change*. Saskatchewan Health, Regina.

Spellbring, A.M. (1991) Nursing's role in health promotion: an overview. *Nursing Clinics of North America*, **26**, 805–14.

Stachtchenko, S. & Jenicek, M. (1990) Conceptual differences between prevention and health promotion: research implications for community health programs. *Canadian Journal of Public Health*, **84**, 53–8.

Tatro, S. & Gleit, C.J. (1983) A wellness model for nursing: promoting high level wellness in any setting through independent nursing functions. *Nursing Leadership*, **6**(1), 5–9.

Taylor, R.B., Ureda, J.R. & Denham, J.W. (1982) *Health Promotion: Principles and Clinical Applications*. Appleton–Century–Crofts, Norwalk, Connecticut.

Townsend, E.A. (1992) Institutional ethnography: explicating the social organization of professional health practices intending client empowerment. *Canadian Journal of Public Health*, **83**(suppl. 1), 558–61.

Webster's Dictionary (1992) *New Webster's Dictionary*. P.S.I. & Associates, Miami, Florida.

Williams, D.M. (1989) Political theory and individualistic health promotion. *Advances in Nursing Science*, **12**(1), 14–25.

WHO (1978) *Primary Health Care: Report of the International Conference on Primary Health Care at Alma-Ata, USSR*, Sept. 6–12, 1978. World Health Organization/UNICEF, Geneva.

WHO (1986) *Health Promotion Concepts and Principles in Action: A Policy Framework*. World Health Organization, Copenhagen.

Chapter 2
Caregivers' emotional wellbeing and their capacity to learn about stroke

VALERIE BRAITHWAITE, PhD

Senior Lecturer, Psychology Department, The Australian National University, Canberra, Australia

and ANNE McGOWN, MA

Lecturer, Psychology Department, Faculty of Science, University of Canberra, Canberra, Australia

This chapter examines the effects of distress on the capacity of informal caregivers of stroke patients to absorb information about stroke and caregiving. Thirty-seven caregivers took part in a stroke seminar. Minor psychiatric symptoms were related to caregivers' knowledge prior to the seminar, with the more emotionally distressed being the least knowledgeable. The emotional state of the caregivers, however, did not affect how much they learnt. Knowledge after the seminar was best predicted from pre-seminar knowledge and age. Older caregivers were less well-informed afterwards, although they did not differ significantly from younger caregivers in their scores initially. These findings do not discount the possibility that emotional carers are too shocked to take in information from hospital staff at the time of admission. The data do demonstrate that, given time to accept the caregiving role, emotional carers are receptive to learning about stroke and the stroke patient's needs.

Home-based care

Home-based care for stroke patients has long been recommended, and increasingly patients are being discharged from hospitals as soon as possible to continue their rehabilitation from home (Bonita *et al.* 1987; Brocklehurst *et al.* 1981; Mulley & Arie 1978; Wade & Hewer 1983; Wright & Robson 1980). Arguments in favour of home care centre on cost containment and effective rehabilitation. Stroke survivors are unlikely to require medical treatment within the hospital so that their occupying a much needed bed is difficult to justify (Mulley & Arie 1978; Wade & Hewer 1983). However, they do need rehabilitation to assist them to resume independent living to the greatest degree possible.

Studies have shown that the skills acquired in a hospital setting do not always apply to the home; sometimes they are not relevant, and sometimes other skills are required (Andrews & Stewart 1979; Brocklehurst *et al.* 1981; Garraway *et al.* 1980; Labi *et al.* 1980). Home rehabilitation is the logical answer to solving these difficulties.

Home care for the stroke survivor, however, is not without problems. Responsibility for care is often transferred to a family member with no previous experience in caring for someone who has had a stroke. In addition, caregivers have their own adjustments to make. Not only must they learn to meet the needs of the stroke survivor, but they must cope with their own fears and anxieties as they are suddenly cut off from their old lifestyle and thrown into another (Bedsworth & Molen 1982; Braithwaite 1990; Brocklehurst *et al.* 1981; Croog & Fitzgerald 1978; O'Keefe & Gilliss 1988; Schulz *et al.* 1988).

Attitudes of family members

The attitudes of family members have a profound effect on patients' reactions to medical regimens, emotional adaptation and rehabilitation (Bedsworth & Molen 1982). Worry and anxiety can result in family members being overprotective, and inadvertently preventing stroke survivors from achieving their full potential after the stroke (Andrews & Stewart 1979; Brocklehurst *et al.* 1981; Kinsella & Duffy 1980; Labi *et al.* 1980).

In studying 18 families of convalescing myocardial infarction patients, Wishnie *et al.* (1971) observed a steady eroding conflict in the families and high anxiety about the patient and about caregiving responsibilities. The authors attributed the conflict to misunderstanding about the nature of the disease and misinterpretation of physician's orders. It is not surprising, therefore, that families have been encouraged to take part in supportive and educational programmes so that they are better prepared for caregiving (Dring 1989; Jarrett 1981; Mongiardi *et al.* 1987; Overs & Belknap 1967; Stone 1987; Stroker 1983; Wright & Robson 1980).

In spite of widespread support for educational and counselling programmes for patients and their families, clients continue to suffer from lack of information in a range of medical contexts (Boreham & Gibson 1978; Gardner & Stewart 1978; Kinsella & Duffy 1980; Mongiardi *et al.* 1987; Shapiro *et al.* 1983; Sosnowitz 1984; Todd & Still 1984; Waitzkin 1985). Client characteristics which have been most often studied in relation to information-giving have been medical (certainty of diagnosis, prognosis) and socio-demographic in nature (socio-economic status, education, age, sex), but some work has suggested that psychological demeanour affects how much clients are told by medical staff.

One such characteristic examined in relation to caregivers is level of emotionality or neurosis: the degree to which a person is observed or self-reports as having low tolerance for stress, emotions which are easily aroused, and a tendency toward symptoms of anxiety and depression (Braithwaite 1987; Eysenck 1967). Those who are unable to control their emotions are perceived by medical staff as being difficult and interactions with them are limited. Explanations for such avoidance vary: the time constraints of medical staff, their feelings of inadequacy, emotional self-protection, a desire to punish inappropriate behaviour, and a belief that clients are not ready to be told or are unable to hear (Bedsworth & Molen 1982; Cassem & Hackett 1972; Lipton & Svarstad 1977; Sosnowitz 1984).

The belief that emotional clients do not retain the information that they are given is particularly threatening to effective rehabilitation programmes. Clinical reports have referred to families as being too anxious to hear what is being said (O'Keefe & Gilliss 1988; Stone 1987). Medical staff who associate poor information retention with emotionality have little incentive to provide information to distressed clients. Yet these are the clients who are purported to be most likely to benefit from greater understanding and knowledge (Dzau & Boehme 1978; Kinsella & Duffy 1980). Emotional carers are likely to be doubly disadvantaged by their psychological state, missing vital information initially and suffering increased anxiety through lack of knowledge.

Stereotyped emotional caregivers

In a recent study, McGown & Braithwaite (1992) found that emotional caregivers were stereotyped as being less able to absorb information than carers showing outward signs of emotional control. Respondents were presented with a series of vignettes describing wives interacting with their husbands and with medical staff after their spouse's stroke. Groups of nurses, caregivers and members of the general public rated each of the vignette wives on five-point rating scales which represented how emotional they considered the wife to be and how capable they thought she was of absorbing information about her husband's condition. While nurses and the general public judged emotional behaviour as a sign that information could not be taken in properly, caregivers themselves made no such inference. Caregivers, furthermore, were more positive than the nurses in their assessment of the wives' capacity to absorb information. Biases against emotional caregivers in medical settings were clearly not shared by the caregivers themselves.

If this bias against emotional caregivers is to be dealt with fairly and sensitively, information is required on how able emotional carers are to absorb information. The adverse effects of anxiety on memory have been well documented experimentally (Kausler 1990), but it would be a mistake to assume that such research translates unproblematically into this setting.

Motivations to help the patient and ensure that the best care is provided are high in the relatives of hospital patients. Distress over the wellbeing of another person may lead to the facilitating effects of anxiety outweighing the debilitating effects, with the family's motivation to know and understand particularly high.

The study

The purpose of this research was to explore the capacity of more emotional caregivers to learn about stroke in an applied setting. As a first step in challenging and questioning biases against emotional relatives, caregivers were recruited for a stroke education seminar. The dependent variable was knowledge gained through the seminar.

Emotionality was operationalized in two ways. First, emotionality was defined in terms of mental wellbeing, or more specifically by symptoms of anxiety and depression. The second definition focused on the caregiving burden and the stress associated with providing care.

Emotionality was reflected in the extent to which caregivers felt inadequate in the caregiving role and were experiencing disruption. Feeling inadequate as a caregiver was considered particularly important because of a possible relationship with Wicklund & Frey's (1980) notion of objective self-awareness. When objectively aware, the individual directs attention inward, evaluating the self, and is not receptive to happenings in the outside world. Carers who express personal inadequacy may be in a state of objective self-awareness, and therefore be unable to take in the information that medical staff have given them about the stroke survivor's condition.

The association between emotionality and knowledge among experienced caregivers is likely to be affected by a third variable, the intensity of care required by the stroke survivor. Well-informed caregivers could be the more emotional caregivers because of the demanding nature of their role and their motivation to meet these demands. In contrast, caregivers with fewer demands may be not only less interested in acquiring information but also less emotional. The demands of caregiving were defined in terms of the functional health of the stroke survivor and in terms of deficits in his or her social and psychological functioning.

Method

Participants

Thirty-seven stroke carers volunteered to take part in the seminar: 28 females and nine males. Because they are not patients, carers were difficult to contact through the traditional health system. This study used snowballing or net-work sampling to contact them; a strategy often used to locate subjects from less accessible groups (Burns & Grove 1987). Stroke clubs were the first point of contact. When interviewed, these volunteers were asked to help the researchers find other stroke carers. While the representativeness of such samples is always open to question, the demographic profile was not dissimilar from that reported in other caregiving studies (Braithwaite 1990), with one exception. The present study had a disproportionately large number of spouse caregivers.

Participants ranged in age from 25 to 78 years (M = 61.11, SD = 10.38), with the majority (62%) being over 60 years of age. Thirty-one were caring for a spouse, five were caring for a parent and one for a parent-in-law. The sample comprised relatively experienced caregivers, all but two being in this role for more than one year. On average, the time that had elapsed since the stroke was 3.78 years (SD = 2.77). Participants were assured that any information they provided would be treated confidentially.

Design

The dependent variable, knowledge about stroke, was assessed by a multiple choice test taken by participants before the seminar and afterwards. The seminar lasted for two hours and covered:

(1) The prevalence of stroke.
(2) Risk factors.
(3) Hospitalization practices.
(4) The treatment of stroke and its effects.
(5) The stresses of caregiving.
(6) Resources available to caregivers.

A lecture format was adopted, interspersed with questions from participants and discussion of issues raised. Seminars were offered at a number of different times to accommodate as many interested caregivers as possible.

The seminar and the multiple choice test were pre-tested on a sample of 26 nurses to ensure that both gave adequate scope for caregivers to demonstrate and improve their knowledge. These data also provided a baseline for interpreting how knowledgeable the caregivers were and how able they were to learn in this setting. It is important to note, however, that the nurses were not representative of the nursing population. They were volunteers from two major hospitals.

Prior to the seminar, caregivers completed a short questionnaire which was appended to the multiple choice test Symptoms of depression and anxiety in the caregiver, caregiving burden, functional disability of the stroke survivor, and psycho-social loss in the stroke survivor were assessed. Background information regarding the caregiver's age and sex, the relationship of caregiver to care recipient, and the elapsed time since the stroke was also collected via the questionnaire.

Measures

Knowledge

The knowledge scale comprised 13 items taken from a 19-question multiple choice test. The items tapped medical knowledge (e.g. risk factors for stroke, the nature of stroke, its treatment, effects and prognosis) and awareness of issues of carer wellbeing. The six items not included in the analysis were either ones which almost all carers were able to answer on the pre-test questionnaire or which were not well intercorrelated with other questions. Each item was scored as correct (1) or incorrect (0). Scores on the knowledge scale at the time of the pre-test were normally distributed and ranged from 0 to 13 with a mean of 6.32 and standard deviation of 2.55. The alpha reliability coefficient for the scale was 0.71.

Symptoms of anxiety and depression

A brief psychiatric screening instrument, the 4-NS (Henderson *et al.* 1981), was used. In this index, four mental health symptoms – anxiety, depression, irritability and nervousness – were embedded in a total list of 15 symptoms which included sore throats, backache, indigestion, palpitations, and so on. The instrument has been used successfully in community studies where an efficient and unobtrusive measure of mental wellbeing was required.

The reliability and validity of the measure has been investigated in community samples and in caregiving samples (Braithwaite 1990; Henderson *et al.* 1981). Henderson *et al.* reported correlations of 0.62 with the PSE (Present State Examination) and 0.52 and 0.58 with the GHQ (General Health Questionnaire), while Braithwaite found that the 4-NS correlated 0.63 with the DSSI/sAD (Delusions-Symptoms-States Inventory) and had an alpha reliability coefficient of 0.70. In this study, scores ranged from 0 to 4 with a mean of 1.22 and standard deviation of 1.24. Thirty-eight per cent of the sample complained of two or more symptoms. The alpha reliability coefficient for the scale was 0.60.

Burden

The stress of caregiving was assessed through a 16-item scale which asked carers the extent to which they felt inadequate, guilty, resentful, disrupted and disadvantaged by the caring experience (Braithwaite 1990). The original scale contained 17 items, but one was excluded because of insufficient variability among this sample of caregivers. The reliability and validity of the scale had been established in two previous studies of caregivers (Braithwaite 1990; Groube 1990). The items were scored in terms of whether they were true for the carer (1) or not (0). Scale scores ranged from 0 to 14 with a mean of 4.89 and a standard deviation of 3.78. The alpha reliability coefficient was 0.82.

The burden scale could be separated into two highly correlated components, inadequacy and disruption. Because of the relevance of feelings of personal inadequacy to the hypothesis, the two subscales were also used separately. The alpha reliability coefficient for the inadequacy scale was 0.78 and for the disruption scale 0.68.

Functional disability

Carers were asked how much assistance they had to provide for the stroke survivor with 11 activities of daily living: eating, dressing, standing and sitting, transferring, walking, toileting, bathing, communicating, organizing, dealing with finances, and making social contacts. Responses were recorded on a three-point scale according to whether assistance was not provided (1), was provided a little (2), or was provided all the time (3). Scale scores ranged from 13 to 33 with a mean of 19.90 and standard deviation of 5.32. The alpha reliability coefficient was 0.86.

Psycho-social loss

The extent to which the care recipient was psychologically and socially disabled was assessed by an eight-item behaviour checklist which tapped mood disturbance and difficulty in relating to others (e.g. goes on and on about certain things, constantly demands assistance, does not understand what is said, gets deeply depressed). Behaviours were checked as present (1) or absent (0). The scale scores ranged from 0 to 7 with a mean of 2.70 and standard deviation of 2.12. The alpha reliability coefficient was 0.70.

Results

Overall participants' post-seminar scores on the knowledge test (M = 8.89, SD = 2.14) were higher than the pre-seminar scores (M = 6.32, SD = 2.55) ($t(36) = 10.28$, $P < 0.001$). Change scores for individuals varied from −1.00 to 7.00 (M = 2.57, SD = 1.52). From Table 2.1, knowledge scores before and after the seminar were not related to the caregiver's sex, the relationship to

Table 2.1 Correlations of emotionality and caregiving characteristics with pre-seminar and post-seminar knowledge and change scores.

	Knowledge		
Variables	Pre	Post	Change
Background			
Sex	0.08	0.15	0.08
Age	−0.16	−0.39**	−0.27
Spouse	0.12	−0.02	−0.22
Time Caring	0.02	−0.11	−0.18
Emotional status			
Symptoms	−0.40**	−0.35*	0.18
Burden	0.00	0.08	0.11
Inadequacy	0.14	0.25	0.11
Disruption	−0.12	−0.08	0.09
Caregiving demands			
Functional disability	0.20	0.06	−0.26
Psycho-social loss	−0.14	−0.02	0.19

* $P < 0.05$; ** $P < 0.01$.

the stroke survivor, or the time that had elapsed since the stroke. The caregiver's age, however, was related to knowledge. Although older carers were not significantly less informed than younger carers prior to the seminar, they were less informed on the post-seminar test ($r = -0.39$, $n = 37$, $P < 0.01$).

The indices of emotionality, symptoms of poor mental health and caregiving burden, correlated with each other as expected ($r = 0.51$, $n = 37$, $P < 0.001$). The symptom measure also correlated with the inadequacy ($r = 0.45$, $n = 37$, $P < 0.01$) and disruption ($r = 0.48$, $n = 37$, $P < 0.001$) subscales. The emotionality indices were not significantly related to the caregiver's age, sex, relationship to the stroke survivor, or the time that had elapsed since the stroke.

As the first stage in testing the hypothesis that emotional caregivers are disadvantaged in learning about stroke, Pearson product-moment correlation coefficients were calculated between the knowledge indices and the emotionality and caregiving demand measures (see Table 2.1). Symptoms of poor mental health were related significantly to both pre-seminar knowledge and post-seminar knowledge. Variables which were specific to caregiving, that is, stress, workload and disability resulting from stroke, did not correlate significantly with either knowledge measure. In particular, carers who felt inadequate were not less well-informed either before or after the seminar. Clearly, inadequacy does not reflect a state of objective self-awareness.

Knowledge

The greater knowledge of caregivers with better mental health after the seminar appears to be more a function of their knowledge initially than of their greater capacity to learn. The low correlation between symptoms and change in knowledge scores is consistent with this interpretation. Another way of examining the effect of symptoms on a caregiver's capacity to learn was through a regression model in which post-seminar knowledge was regressed on symptoms of poor mental health, once the pre-seminar knowledge of the caregivers was controlled. This strategy was considered preferable to using change in knowledge scores because it avoided the problem of increasing the error term in the dependent variable with a relatively small sample. Also included as a control variable in the regression model was the caregiver's age.

From Table 2.2, the major predictors of knowledge after the seminar were age and pre-seminar knowledge. Those who were younger and who were better informed initially were more likely to be more knowledgeable after the seminar. Of importance is the finding that minor psychiatric symptoms, the major correlate of pre-seminar knowledge, did not contribute to explaining the gains in knowledge made during the seminar.

Table 2.2   Beta coefficients and R^2 values for a hierarchical regression analysis predicting post-seminar knowledge.

	Post-seminar knowledge	
Predictors	Model 1	Model 2
Age	−0.26*	−0.25*
Pre-knowledge	0.77***	0.73***
Symptoms		−0.12
R^2	0.73***	0.74***
Change R^2		0.01

*$P < 0.05$; **$P < 0.01$; ***$P < 0.001$.

These data suggest that emotionally unstable carers are as capable of learning about stroke as those who are emotionally stable. Such an inference needs to be made with caution because it involves accepting the null hypothesis in a situation where the statistical test has low power. An interesting question to ask in conjunction with this conclusion, therefore, is whether or not emotional caregivers improved on their pre-seminar score as much as unemotional caregivers. Two subgroups of carers were formed: those without any symptoms and those who reported two or more symptoms prior to the seminar. The mean knowledge scores of carers without symptoms changed from 7.47 to 9.87 over the course of the seminar, a 2.4 difference ($t(14)=6.87$, $P < 0.001$). The mean for carers with two or more symptoms changed from 5.50 to 8.14, a difference of 2.6 ($t(13)=7.10$, $P < 0.001$). For this group of caregivers, knowledge acquisition was not sacrificed because of their feelings of anxiety and depression.

Comparison group

Practical constraints militated against the use of a control group in this study, leaving unanswered the question of whether change in a caregiver's scores reflected a better understanding of stroke or a 'practice effect'. Some insight into this problem can be gleaned from a comparison of the pre-and post-test scores of the 26 nurses who had volunteered for the pilot study (Table 2.3). No significant change was observed in this group, suggesting that the gain of the caregivers was more likely to represent information than methodological artefact.

Table 2.3   Comparison of carer and nurse knowledge scores before and after stroke seminar.

Knowledge	n	M	SD	t
Pre-seminar				
Carers	37	6.32	2.55	−3.40**
Nurses	26	8.11	1.63	
Post-seminar				
Carers	37	8.89	2.14	0.09
Nurses	26	8.84	1.71	

**$P < 0.01$.

A further question which can be answered from these data is how well informed carers were initially. The knowledge of a professional group such as nurses provides a useful benchmark for addressing the question. The scores of the 16 nurses who have completed the multiple choice knowledge test in the pilot study were compared with those of carers before and after the seminar (Table 2.3). Nurses scored significantly higher than carers on the test before the seminar. A comparison of nurse and carer scores after the seminar produced no significant differences in their knowledge of stroke and caregiving.

Discussion

This study examined the capacity of caregivers to learn about stroke and the extent to which those who were more emotionally distressed were handicapped in their acquisition and recall of knowledge. Previous research has suggested that families may be provided with less information than they would like because medical staff doubt their capacity to absorb information, particularly when they are emotionally unstable.

Emotionality was defined in this study in terms of caregiver stress and symptoms. Both are considered appropriate indicators of emotional instability in experienced caregivers. These data provide no evidence of either psychological state hindering caregivers in their quest for knowledge. Before elaborating further on the findings, however, two limitations imposed by the sample need to be acknowledged. First, the carers who participated in this study had settled into the caring role. The sampling strategy did not provide the researchers with access to families of stroke survivors at the time of hospitalization or of a medical diagnosis. Second, the carers who took part were volunteers, and as such were probably keen to improve their knowledge and understanding of stroke.

The gains in knowledge accomplished by this group of caregivers were not inconsequential. By the end of the seminar, the mean knowledge score for caregivers equalled that of nurses who had been caring for stroke patients. These data suggest that the capacities of caregivers, particularly emotional caregivers, may be underestimated by nursing and medical staff.

Differences in information gain

At the same time, differences did exist in this group in how easily information was assimilated and in how knowledgeable caregivers were initially. Older caregivers had more difficulty with the seminar than others. Although their knowledge scores increased significantly as a group (from 5.33 to 7.60 for those aged 65 and over) ($t(14) = 5.72$, $P < 0.001$), older carers showed less of a gain than those who were younger. This result is a reminder that presentation style and pace should be modified to suit the age group, and that consultation with the group about preferred presentation styles is appropriate and efficient in the long term.

The second important finding was that, although carers with minor psychiatric symptoms were not disadvantaged in the course of the seminar, they were less knowledgeable initially. This result is consistent with the underlying rationale of the study, that medical staff underestimate the informational capacity of caregivers. Nevertheless, an alternative explanation must be seriously considered. Symptoms of poor mental health may not pre-date the medical staff's sharing of knowledge with families, but rather be a consequence of inadequate knowledge. For whatever reason, some families may not be provided with information at the time of the stroke and may fail to open channels of communication themselves. As a consequence of their ignorance, their emotional well-being may suffer.

The seriousness of this problem is well recognized in the medical literature. According to Stedeford (1981), 'Poor communication causes more suffering than any other problem except unrelieved pain'.

While this interpretation cannot be rejected, it is made less plausible by what we know of the association between symptoms of anxiety and depression and having an emotional temperament. Depression and anxiety have been linked not only to life events, but also to personality dispositions, in particular, neuroticism (Braithwaite 1987; Costa & McCrae 1980; Eysenck 1967; Eysenck & Eysenck 1969; Henderson *et al.* 1981). It is likely that depressed and anxious caregivers have temperaments of the kind that would lead them to be also highly emotional at the time of the stroke crisis. Their emotionality at this stage is likely to be linked with their missing out on important information.

Emotional caregivers

If emotional caregivers miss out on information at the time of the stroke crisis, is the problem one of not being told or not being able to comprehend what they are told? It is tempting to infer from these data that the problem is one of not being told. Such a conclusion assumes that the emotionality carers experience in the caregiving role is comparable to that which they experience in the crisis situation. This may not be the case. At the time of the stroke, emotionality may involve shock, passivity and self-protection; a shutting down response to avoid further threatening information. This is consistent with clinical descriptions of carers as shocked, numb, and unable to comprehend or make decisions in the early stages of the illness (Kinsella & Duffy 1980; O'Keefe & Gillis 1988).

When the responsibility for care is transferred to family carers, emotionality may be no longer an expression of shock, but rather of responsibility, dread and worry about what to do. In this state, carers may be aware of their need for information and be more receptive to those who are willing and able to provide it. Although this qualification of the data is speculative, it offers the advantage of accommodating disparate clinical observations and research findings.

Conclusion

Whether or not the emotionality of carers in the crisis situation can be shown to be functionally different from emotionality in the caregiving role is a question for future research. In the meantime, successful intervention with stroke survivors may be increased by the adoption of a more dynamic conception of caregivers' needs. The challenge facing nursing and medical staff is to recognize the right time for providing information.

These data demonstrate that the stigmatizing of emotional carers as being unable to absorb information is unjustified. They may initially forget what they have been told. They may irritate staff by repeating the same question and making unrealistic demands. But after they have had time to adjust to their new role, emotional carers can become more knowledgeable about stroke. Heightened emotionality need no impair capacity to learn.

Acknowledgements

The authors wish to thank the Department of Psychology, The Australian National University, and the Buehler Center for Aging, Northwestern University, for their support for this project.

References

Andrews, K. & Stewart J. (1979) Stroke recovery: he can but does he? *Rheumatology and Rehabilitation*, **18**, 43–8.
Bedsworth, J.A. & Molen, M.J. (1982) Psychological stress in spouses of patients with myocardial infarction. *Heart and Lung*, **11**, 450–56.
Bonita, R., Anderson, A. & North, J.D.K. (1987) The pattern of management after stroke. *Age and Ageing*, **16**, 29–34.
Boreham, P. & Gibson, D. (1978) The informative process in private medical consultations: a preliminary investigation. *Social Science and Medicine*, **12**, 409–16.
Braithwaite, V.A. (1987) The Scale of Emotional Arousability: bridging the gap between the neuroticism construct and its measurement. *Psychological Medicine*, **17**, 217–25.
Braithwaite, V.A. (1990) *Bound to Care*. Allen & Unwin, Sydney.
Brocklehurst, J.C., Morris, P., Andrews, K., Richards, B. & Laycock, P. (1981) Social effects of stroke. *Social Science and Medicine*, **15A**, 35–9.
Burns, N. & Grove, S.K. (1987) *The Practice of Nursing Research: Conduct, Critique and Utilization*. W.B. Sanders, Philadelphia.
Cassem, N. & Hackett, T. (1972) Sources of tension for the CCU nurse. *American Journal of Nursing*, **72**, 1426–30.
Costa, P.T. Jr & McCrae, R.R. (1980) Still stable after all these years: personality as a key to some issues in adulthood and old age. In *Life-Span Development and Behavior*, vol. 3 (Eds P.B. Baltes & D.G. Brim Jr), pp. 65–101. Academic Press, New York.
Croog, S.H. & Fitzgerald, E.F. (1978) Subjective stress and serious illness of a spouse: wives of heart patients. *Journal of Health and Social Behavior*, **19**, 166–78.
Dring, R. (1989) The informal caregiver responsible for home care of the individual with cognitive dysfunction following brain injury. *Journal of Neuroscience*, **21**, 42–5.
Dzau, R.E. & Boehme, A.R. (1978) Stroke rehabilitation: a family-team education program. *Archives of Physical Medicine and Rehabilitation*, **59**, 236–9.
Eysenck, H.J. (1967) *Biological Basis of Personality*. C.C. Thomas, Springfield, Illinois.
Eysenck, H.J. & Eysenck, S.B.G. (1969) *Personality Structure and Measurement*. R.R. Knapp, San Diego, California.
Gardner, D. & Stewart, N. (1978) Staff involvement with families of patients in critical-care units. *Heart & Lung*, **7**, 105–10.
Garraway, W.M., Akhtar, A.J., Prescott, R.J. & Hockey, L. (1980) Management of acute stroke in the elderly: preliminary results of a controlled trial. *British Medical Journal*, **280**, 1040–43.

40 *Nursing Care of Adults*

Groube, M. (1990) Stress, social support and adaptation among caregivers. Master of Clinical Psychology Thesis. The Australian National University, Canberra.

Henderson, A.S., Byrne, D.G. & Duncan-Jones, P. (1981) *Neurosis and the Social Environment.* Academic Press, Sydney.

Jarrett, S.R. (1981) Stroke patient: home or hospital? *Lancet*, i, 46.

Kausler, D.H. (1990) Motivation, human aging, and cognitive performance. In *Handbook of the Psychology of Aging*, 3rd edn (Eds J.E. Birren & K. Warner Schaie), pp. 171–182. Academic Press, San Diego, California.

Kinsella, G.J. & Duffy, F.D. (1980) Attitudes towards disability expressed by spouses of stroke patients. *Scandinavian Journal of Rehabilitation Medicine*, 12, 73–6.

Labi, M.L.C., Phillips, T.F. & Gresham, G.E. (1980) Psychosocial disability in physically restored long-term stroke survivors. *Archives of Physical Medicine and Rehabilitation*, 61, 561–5.

Lipton, H.L. & Svarstad, B. (1977) Sources of variation in clinicians' communication to parents about mental retardation. *American Journal of Mental Deficiency*, 82, 155–61.

McGown, A. & Braithwaite, V. (1992) Stereotypes of emotional caregivers and their capacity to absorb information: the views of nurses, stroke carers and the general public. *Journal of Advanced Nursing*, 17(7), 822–8.

Mongiardi, F., Payman, B.C. & Hawthorn, P.J (1987) The needs of relatives of patients admitted to the coronary care unit. *Intensive Care Nursing*, 3, 67–70.

Mulley, G. & Arie, T. (1978) Treating stroke: home or hospital? *British Medical Journal*, ii(11 November), 1321–2.

O'Keefe, B. & Gilliss, C.L. (1988) Family care in the coronary care unit: an analysis of clinical nurse specialist intervention. *Heart & Lung*, 17, 191–8.

Overs, R.P. & Belknap, E.L. (1967) Educating stroke patient families. *Journal of Chronic Disease*, 20, 45–51.

Schulz, R., Tompkins, C.A. & Rau, M.T. (1988) A longitudinal study of the psychosocial impact of stroke on primary support persons. *Psychology and Aging*, 3, 131–41.

Shapiro, M.C., Bill, F., Joe, A., Smith, C., Fred, C., Bruce, C. *et al.* (1983) Information control and the exercise of power in the obstetrical encounter. *Social Science and Medicine*, 17, 139–46.

Sosnowitz, B.G. (1984) Managing parents on neonatal intensive care units. *Social Problems*, 31, 390–402.

Stedeford, A. (1981) Couples facing death II. Unsatisfactory communication. *British Medical Journal*, 283, 1098–101.

Stone, S.P. (1987) The Mount Vernon Stroke Service: a feasibility study to determine whether it is possible to apply the principles of stroke unit management to patients and their families on general medical wards. *Age and Ageing*, 16, 81–8.

Stroker, R. (1983) Impact of disability on families of stroke clients. *Journal of Neurosurgical Nursing*, 15, 360–65.

Todd, C.J. & Still, A.W. (1984) Communication between general practitioners and patients dying at home. *Social Science and Medicine*, 18, 667–72.

Wade, D.T. & Hewer, R.L. (1983) Why admit stroke patients to hospital? *Lancet*, i(9 April), 807–9.

Waitzkin, H. (1985) Information giving in medical care. *Journal of Health and Social Behavior*, 26, 81–101.

Wickland, R.A. & Frey, D. (1980) Self-awareness theory: when the self makes a difference. In *The Self in Social Psychology* (Eds D.M. Wegner & R.R. Vallacher), pp. 31–54. Oxford University Press, New York.

Wishnie, H., Hackett, R. & Cassem, N. (1971) Psychological hazards of convalescence following myocardial infarction. *Journal of the American Medical Association*, 215, 1292–6.

Wright, W.B. & Robson, P. (1980) Crisis procedure for stroke at home. *Lancet*, ii(2 August), 249.

Chapter 3
Monitoring the pressure sore problem in a teaching hospital

CAROL DEALEY, BSc(Hons), SRN, RCNT

Clinical Nurse Specialist in Tissue Viability, Community Hospitals Division,
Southern Birmingham Community Health NHS Trust, Birmingham, England

During 1989 and 1990 a series of three prevalence surveys were undertaken in a West Midlands teaching hospital to identify the numbers of patients at risk of developing pressure sores and the actual number of patients with pressure sores, prior to the purchase of pressure relieving equipment. A further survey was undertaken in January 1993 to examine any improvement in pressure sore prevention strategies and in the care of those with established pressure sores. All in-patients were assessed using the Waterlow score. Full details of all pressure sores and any pressure relieving equipment in use was recorded. The findings were compared with those of the first survey in 1989. The prevalence for 1989 was 8.77%, and this had reduced slightly to 7.9% in 1993. There was no significant difference in these figures. However, in 1989 35 patients had 64 pressure sores and in 1993 32 patients had 46 pressure sores. There was a significant reduction in the actual numbers of pressure sores. There was no significant difference in the grades of sores and the sacrum was the most frequent position in both surveys. The survey showed an improvement in the management of established pressure sores. There was little change in the patient populations with respect to the degree of risk of pressure sore development. Using the Waterlow score, the numbers of patients found to be in the no risk, at risk, high risk and very high risk categories remained remarkably stable. These surveys will continue to provide a basis for selecting pressure relieving equipment. Measurement of pressure sore incidence is needed in the future to monitor the efficacy of the prevention programme.

Introduction

Pressure sores are a costly problem. They cause distress and increased morbidity to the sufferer and are a drain on scarce resources within the

British National Health Service. The cost to the health service of treating pressure sores has been estimated to be from £60 million to £300 million each year (Lancet 1973; Waterlow 1988). Doubt can be cast over the accuracy of these figures but a very accurate ꞈtudy by Hibbs (1988a) costed the care of one patient with a deep sacral prₑssure sore to be £25 905.58. She also considered the opportunity costs and demonstrated that the money and time spent treating the patient in the study was equivalent to the cost of 17 hip or knee replacements. This study clearly demonstrates how pressure sores can result in considerable expenditure and extended hospital stay.

Hibbs (1988b) has suggested that as many as 95% of these sores could be prevented. Many areas are developing pressure sore prevention policies. Overall preventative measures can be beneficial, especially when vigorously supported by the management team. Any prevention plan should incorporate a method of monitoring pressure sores. Regular prevalence surveys can be used to provide information on the effectiveness of prevention strategies.

The research problem

Following a series of pressure sore prevalence surveys during 1989 and 1990 at a teaching hospital (where medical students receive clinical experience), in the West Midlands, England (Dealey 1991), monies had been made available for the purchase of pressure relieving equipment (hereafter described as support systems). The aim of this study was to establish any improvement in pressure sore prevention strategies and in the care of those patients with established pressure sores.

Review of the literature

There is a vast amount of literature on the subject of pressure sores. The literature was reviewed retrospectively as far back as 1975 because the wealth of material from that date onwards provided plenty of scope for review.

Several policy documents have been published which have a relevance to pressure sore prevention (Royal College of Physicians 1986; Audit Commission 1991; Panel for the Prediction and Prevention of Pressure Ulcers in Adults 1992; Department of Health 1992). These reports all state the importance of pressure sore prevention. They also highlight the need for more information to be obtained on the size of the pressure sore problem generally and the need for accurate, comparable data. They provide support for the relevance of prevalence surveys in any and every health care setting as a means of obtaining information for future planning.

In the past both the nursing and medical professions have laid the blame for pressure sores on 'bad nursing'. Anthony (1989) suggests that nurses can be extremely critical of each other and reluctant to admit the existence of any sores. Dealey (1992a) suggests that in the rush to cast blame on others it is easy to neglect discovering the precise cause of the injury.

The importance of each health authority developing a prevention policy is stressed by Hibbs (1988b) and Livesley & Simpson (1989). Livesley & Simpson (1993) have produced guidelines for developing a prevention strategy which emphasizes the importance of the multidisciplinary team. The particular importance of the nurse's role in prevention is discussed by Dealey (1989). Whilst nurses have their responsibilities, so do the medical staff. Bliss (1988) suggests that pressure sores are not the result of 'bad nursing', but the failure of a doctor to recognize the vulnerability of acutely ill or newly paralysed patients.

Methodologies used

Review of the methodologies used by other researchers when undertaking surveys is a useful stating point when designing a survey. Many have been undertaken, most as a point prevalence survey, a 'snap shot' taken on a single day. Such a survey was undertaken by Clark *et al.* (1978) in the Greater Glasgow Health Authority, Scotland. Both hospital and community patients were included. The data were collected by means of a questionnaire. The results showed that 8.8% of the patients surveyed had pressure sores. Spot checks found that there was confusion over the definition of grade 1 sores and so they were all excluded from the findings; the reliability of the other gradings was satisfactory. (Grade 1 sores were defined as skin discoloration or erythema (redness) which does not fade when pressure is removed.)

The survey by Ek & Boman (1982) used a different methodology, that of interviewing nurses on all the wards in the public health services area in Sweden during a one-week period. No grading system was used to describe the sores. A 4% prevalence was found.

The largest survey undertaken in this country was that by David *et al.* (1983). Hospital patients in 20 health districts within four health regions were surveyed. The data were collected by means of a structured interview. A grading system was used to describe the scores. The overall prevalence was found to be 6.7%.

Warner & Hall (1986) undertook a survey in one hospital. Data were collected on the same day for four consecutive weeks. Details were recorded of the site and grades of the pressure sores. The prevalence of sores was 14%. Nyquist & Hawthorn (1987) surveyed a health authority. The data were collected by means of two questionnaires. The patient's Norton score was calculated and the sores were graded and measured. Tests for reliability were not reported. The prevalence rate was found to be 5.3%.

Clark & Cullum (1992) reported on a series of prevalence surveys carried out in one health district over a four-year period. Details were collected as to whether a patient was admitted with a sore or developed a sore on the current ward. They report a prevalence of 6.8% in the first survey and 14.2% in the final year.

Meehan (1992) reported on a multi-site prevalence survey carried out in the USA. The grade and position of pressure sores was recorded as well as details of any support systems. Observations were carried out on 34 987 patients of whom 3230 had pressure sores, giving a national prevalence of 9.2%.

O'Dea (1993) found a much higher prevalence than other surveys. She surveyed a total of 3213 patients and had a prevalence of 18.6%. Again the accuracy of grade 1 sores was questioned.

Accuracy of data

Several studies highlight the difficulty in collecting accurate data (Warner & Hall 1986; Ibbotson 1988; Ling & Vincent 1989). Warner & Hall suggest that whilst reports of sores are likely to be accurate, the reports of no sores may be an over-estimate. This may be due to lack of knowledge by the person completing the form or it may be due to a reluctance to declare the existence of sores. Ibbotson (1988) found that there was a discrepancy between a survey of patient records during the day and the numbers of pressure sores reported by the night staff. She suggested that this may have been due to some confusion in recognizing grade 1 sores.

The difficulty of recognizing grade 1 sores has already been noted. It is important to consider the methods of grading sores so that the most reliable might be selected. Most grading systems seem to be fairly similar. They all work on the premise that the higher the grade, the deeper the sore. Johnson (1985) suggested a five grade system and provided colour photographs to illustrate each grade. This is a useful way of ensuring effective communication. The draft National Clinical Guidelines for Pressure Sore Management and Prevention suggest that grade 1 sores should not be included when documenting pressure sore prevalence and incidence (NHSE 1995). Future surveys will take note of this.

There are also a number of risk assessment scoring systems. The purpose of these scoring systems is to provide a simple method of identifying those at risk of pressure sore development. The earliest scoring system to be developed was the Norton score (Norton *et al.* 1975). Currently, the most widely used scoring system in the United Kingdom is the Waterlow score (Waterlow 1985). This may be because it is seen to be relevant to a wider range of patients.

The study

The overall design for this empirical study was a time series design using comparative surveys. A survey is defined as descriptive research where a situation or area of interest is accurately and systematically described (Isaacs & Michael 1981). However, a comparative survey falls into the category of quasi-experimental research. In this type of research there is an approximate of the experimental design, but it is undertaken in conditions where it is not possible to control of manipulate all the variables.

Population

The population that was studied was all in-patients in a teaching hospital on the days of the surveys. The dependent variable was pressure sores which were very clearly defined using the following operational definitions.

(1) A pressure sore is damage to the skin caused by pressure, shear or friction or a combination of any of these.
(2) Pressure sores were graded in the following way.
Grade 1: redness which does not fade and blanches under light pressure.
Grade 2: redness which does not blanch, blistering or superficial break in the skin.
Grade 3: break in the skin through to the dermis.
Grade 4: sore down to the subcuticular layer.
Grade 5: sore extends to other tissue, e.g. muscle, tendon or bone.

Prevalence surveys

A pressure sore point prevalence survey which was carried out in 1989 provided the necessary information for the initial survey.

The 1989 survey was intended to provide guidance on the type of pressure relieving equipment that was needed for the patient population within the hospital. The method of data collection was intended to avoid some of the problems found by other researchers. The investigator attended a nurses' meeting to explain the value of collecting the data. A link nurse from each ward or unit had overall responsibility for the data collection in their areas.

A series of meetings were held to provide standardized information about the survey. In particular, the Waterlow score, which was to be used to assess the degree of risk of pressure sore development for all patients, was explained. Colour photographs of each grade of pressure sore were provided for each area. Details of the Waterlow score, presence of pressure sores and the use of special mattresses or beds were collected for each patient. Further details were collected with respect to those patients with pressure sores, concerning the position, grade and treatment of the sore. Whilst the survey measured overall prevalence of pressure sores, those patients admitted with sores are identified so that they could be subtracted from the total if desired.

A further point prevalence survey was carried out in 1993 using the same methodology as the original survey. As this survey had identified the degree of risk of pressure sore development of all the patients, it was easy to identify any changes in the current patient population. A serious alteration in population would have invalidated the findings.

Information obtained

The following information was obtained and used to compare the two surveys:

(1) The size of the total patient population.
(2) The prevalence of pressure sores.
(3) The numbers of patients admitted with pressure sores.
(4) The numbers of pressure sores which developed after admission.
(5) The position and grade of the sores.
(6) The treatment of the sores.
(7) The progress of the sores.
(8) The range of support systems in use.
(9) The degree of risk of pressure sore development in all the patients.
(10) Analysis of the Waterlow scores of all patients with pressure sores.

Results

Numbers of patients with pressure sores

The total number of in-patients in the hospital during both surveys did not vary greatly. The number of patients with pressure sores was slightly lower in the 1993 survey than in the 1989 survey. The numbers were as follows:

1989 survey: 399 patients of whom 35 had pressure sores = 8.77%;
1993 survey: 406 patients of whom 32 had pressure sores = 7.9%.

The prevalence data were compared using a chi-squared test. No significant difference was found.

The Waterlow scores of the patients with pressure sores were categorized into the at risk, high risk and very high risk categories for each survey. The findings were similar. In each survey those with pressure sores were found to fall predominantly in the very high risk category in each survey.

Where the pressure sore occurred

The data did not provide information as to the possible causes of the pressure sores, but it did identify when and where the sores occurred. In the 1989 survey this information was only provided on 32 of the 35 patients with sores.

Eighteen patients developed pressure sores during their stay on the ward. A further three patients were transferred from elsewhere in the hospital with existing pressure sores. Of the remaining 11 patients who were admitted to the hospital with pressure sores, five came from home and six came from other hospitals. Thus, 65.6% of sores had occurred in the hospital and 34.4% had occurred elsewhere.

The 1993 survey found that 19 of the patients developed pressure sores during their stay in the ward. A further four patients were transferred from elsewhere in the hospital with existing pressure sores. Of the remaining nine patients who were admitted to the hospital with pressure sores, six were admitted from home and three were admitted from other hospitals. Therefore, 71.9% of the pressure sores occurred in the hospital and 28.1% had occurred elsewhere. There is no statistical difference between the two surveys.

Numbers of pressure sores

In the 1989 survey several patients had more than one pressure sore, so that the 35 patients had a total of 64 sores. This amounted to an average of 1.8 pressure sores per patient. In the 1993 survey the 32 patients had a total of 46 pressure sores which was an average of 1.4 per patient. These numbers were compared using a chi-squared test and there was found to be a significant reduction in the number of pressure sores in the 1993 survey ($P=0.05$).

Grade of the pressure sores

Table 3.1 shows the results for the two surveys. As can be seen there is a difference between the two surveys. Using a chi-squared test, each grade of pressure sore was assessed for any differences between the two surveys. A significant difference was found between the numbers of grade 3 pressure sores, with an increase in the numbers in the later survey ($P=0.05$). Grades 1,

Table 3.1 The grades of pressure sores.

	1989		1993	
Grade	Number	%	Number	%
1	24	37.5	11	23.9
2	25	39.1	15	32.6
3	7	10.9	14	30.4
4	3	4.7	4	8.7
5	5	7.8	2	4.4
Total	64	100	46	100

2 and 3 can be described as less severe sores. If the numbers of these grades are added together and a percentage calculated for each survey it can be seen that there is very little difference, being 87.5% for 1989 and 87% for 1993. The same is obviously true for the severe pressure sores. However, there are less grade 5 sores and more grade 4 sores in 1993 than there were in 1989. The numbers are too small for statistical analysis so it is not possible to judge if there is any significant difference.

Position of the pressure sores

The major difference between the two surveys is the reduction in the number of heel sores, 12 (18.8%) in 1989 and three (6.5%) in 1993. However, the figures are too small for statistical analysis. In both surveys the sacrum was the commonest position for pressure sores, 42.1% and 56.5% respectively.

Treatments being used

There was some difference in the types of dressings being used between the two surveys. However, for both surveys the commonest treatment was actually no dressing. In each survey seven different types of treatment were being used, the range varying each time. The findings for each survey are listed in Table 3.2. No attempt has been made to statistically analyse these treatments.

Table 3.2   The range of treatments being used.

Dressing	1989	1993
None	39	14
Opsite	7	4
Granuflex	6	12
Betadine spray	6	—
Sorbsan	4	6
Silastic foam + Betadine	1	—
Mepore	1	—
Granuflex Extra Thin	—	5
Lyofoam	—	4
Intrasite Gel	—	1
Total	64	46

Progress of the sores

The progress of the sores was not recorded on every patient in either survey. In the first survey the progress of 15 patients was described as static whereas only eight were so described in 1993. In 1989, eight were described as deteriorating and seven were improving. In 1993, 12 patients had an improvement in their pressure sores and five were deteriorating. In the case of two patients in each survey the respondent was not sure of the progress of the sore. This was usually because the patient had recently been admitted to the ward or unit.

Pressure relieving equipment

The researcher already had a fairly accurate estimate of the equipment within the hospital. At the time of the first survey, there was very little available and 21 patients with pressure sores were not on any type of pressure relieving device. Since 1990 a number of support systems were purchased and distributed to wards according to the needs highlighted by the surveys in 1989 and 1990. In the 1993 survey only four patients with pressure sores were not provided with a support system.

Degree of risk of pressure sore development in the hospital population

The Waterlow score can be used to divide patients into one of four categories: no risk, at risk, high risk and very high risk. The data from each of the surveys were collated to place all the patients in one of these categories. The numbers for each survey were compared in each of the four categories. The percentage for each category was as follows:

No risk	1989 = 47.9%	
	1993 = 49%	
At risk	1989 = 21.1%	
	1993 = 23.4%	
High risk	1989 = 15.5%	
	1993 = 15%	
Very high risk	1989 = 15.5%	
	1993 = 12.6%	

Using a chi-squared test the results from each survey were compared for the four categories. There was no significant difference between the patients in the two surveys.

Factors of relevance to tissue breakdown

A breakdown of the components of the Waterlow score was recorded for those patients with pressure sores. The individual scores were compared to see which (if any) factors were frequently given high scores. Several factors appeared to be relevant. Those which occurred in more than 10 patients were:

below average weight, bed/chair-bound, over 65 years, tissue malnutrition, neurological deficit and major surgery.

Discussion

Numbers of patients with pressure sores

The prevalence of pressure sores was within the range reported by David *et al.* (1983) for both surveys. It was a source of disappointment that there was not a greater reduction in the numbers of patients with pressure sores between 1989 and 1993. However, other investigators, such as Clark & Cullum (1992) have actually found an increase in the number of pressure sores. It should also be noted that the surveys by O'Dea (1993) found a prevalence of 18.6%, considerably higher than in this survey.

There were a total of 67 patients with pressure sores in the two surveys. The Waterlow score correctly identified as being at risk all but one patient, a sensitivity of 98–9%. Warner & Hall (1986) found that the Norton score had a sensitivity of 65%. This study shows that the Waterlow score would seem to be a more sensitive scoring system than the Norton and certainly more appropriate for the acutely ill patient. A limitation is that there is no record of the Waterlow score at the time the pressure sore occurred.

Nursing workload and levels of staff must also be considered. A recent survey by the Royal College of Nursing (1993) has shown that increased workload and reduced numbers of staff may be seen across the UK. The survey also found that two-thirds of nurses believed that the numbers of qualified staff had fallen and linked this to a lowering of the quality of care they were able to provide. As the presence of pressure sores is often used as a marker for measuring quality of care, it may be that it should be seen as pleasing that the number of patients with pressure sores had not actually increased.

A further factor must be considered: the state of the standard hospital mattresses. Surveys had shown that many mattresses in the hospital were in need of replacement because the foam was collapsed, resulting in grounding. Although some new mattresses had been purchased, funding for a replacement programme had only been obtained at the end of 1992. Whilst there was an improvement in the mattress stock in 1993 compared with 1989, there were still a number of sub-standard mattresses within the hospital. It is impossible to judge whether this had any effect on the development of pressure sores, but it must be considered

Where the sore occurred

Although approximately 30% of patients in each survey were admitted with pressure sores, it must be remembered that the remainder occurred in hospital. Future prevention plans should be looking to reduce this number drastically. This would entail trying to pinpoint the actual time of tissue damage. It may also be appropriate to review equipment such as operating and X-ray tables, as many patients undergo lengthy operations or investigations.

Grade and position of sores

A weakness in the methodology for both the surveys was that there was no system for checking the accuracy of the information collected. Previous studies had shown that there could be difficulty in recognizing grade 1 sores (Clark *et al.* 1978; David *et al.* 1983). Time constraints prevented a system of random checking of data collection. However, the researcher had previously examined some of the patients with sores and so was able to confirm the data on those patients.

It came as no surprise that the sacrum was the commonest position for pressure sores in both surveys. The survey by David *et al.* (1983) and report by Lockett (1983) also found more pressure sores on the sacrum than elsewhere on the body. However, this study found a higher proportion of sacral sores (56.5%) than the numbers reported by Lockett (31%). This is probably because the hospital under investigation is a teaching hospital and the patients are largely acutely ill. The pressure sores found in the survey were from lying rather than sitting. Lockett was reporting on data collected across 20 health authorities which would have included the chronically sick as well as the acutely ill.

Treatments being used

The commonest treatment that was used in either survey was no dressing. Although this is perfectly acceptable for all grade 1 and grade 2 sores where there is no break in the skin, it is not for deeper sores. It was, therefore, cause for concern that three grade 3 sores and one grade 4 sore in the first survey had no dressing. Not only would this have increased the risk of wound infection, but it would also have delayed healing. This may have accounted for the lack of progress towards healing shown in some of the patients, although it must be recognized that the general condition of the patient is also a factor. In the 1993 survey only grade 1 and 2 pressure sores were left exposed. This can be seen as an improvement in the care of these wounds.

The range of dressings had also altered between the two surveys. In particular in 1993 betadine spray was no longer used. This product had been used ritualistically as there is no evidence to support its use on superficial pressure sores. The investigator made an assessment of the dressings being used in both surveys in relation to the grade and position of the pressure sores and any comments made by the nurse. There was a definite improvement in the selection of dressings in 1993 compared with 1989. Nurses seemed to be making a more appropriate choice of dressing that would meet the needs of the individual. The researcher was also pleased to note that all the products being used in 1993 were ones listed in the hospital formulary.

Pressure relieving equipment

In 1989 the hospital possessed very little equipment. Since 1990 there had been a purchasing programme for support systems. Each ward or unit had several static systems appropriate to their type of patients. A variety of alternating pressure air mattresses had also been purchased which were for general use in the hospital.

The 1993 survey showed a greater awareness of the equipment available. Several comments were made about lack of suitable support systems for individual patients. However, four patients with pressure sores had no support system and 13 patients who were shown not to be at risk of developing pressure sores were lying on static systems. A comment made about one patient stated that his Waterlow score had previously been higher. Many patients are often reluctant to part with mattress toppers which they often find more comfortable than the hospital mattress alone.

It has been the aim of the investigator to plan the methodical purchase and maintenance of a range of support systems suitable for the needs of the patient population of the hospital. However, it is difficult to make equipment selection based on research. Young (1992) discussed the need for more research into the many support systems that are available. The selection of products by the investigator has been based on information from laboratory trials, small scale evaluations and discussions with both patients and nurses. Some items have been found to be unsatisfactory and replaced with alternatives. Thus, an attempt has been made to base selection of support systems on the current level of understanding, albeit limited, and the degree of risk of pressure sore development in the hospital population.

Many writers have proposed the need for an adequate supply of pressure relieving mattresses to assist in pressure sore prevention (Royal College of Physicians 1986; Hibbs 1988a; Livesley & Simpson 1993). Clark & Cullum (1992) have warned against the uncontrolled purchase of support systems. However, they do not suggest what might be used to reduce the numbers of pressure sores. Perhaps education is the most important factor. If staff understand the assessment of patients and appropriate targeting of equipment as well as its usage, there will be a reduction in the numbers of pressure sores (Dealey 1992b). The findings of this study suggest that whilst there is improvement in the numbers of support systems available, there is a need to provide improved staff education in their usage.

Degree of risk of pressure sore development in the hospital population

It was interesting to see that the patient population had not altered greatly in 1993 from that of 1989. Any major alteration would have meant that the two surveys could not be compared with any validity. However, this was not the case. This stability in the pressure sore risk of the hospital population gave support to the investigator's thesis that it is reasonable to select support systems based on the results of prevalence surveys. The value of recording the degree of risk of pressure sore development using a risk calculator can also be seen.

Factors of relevance to tissue breakdown

Some of the factors identified as being relevant to the development of pressure sores were also seen in other studies. One example is age. Pressure sores are frequently associated with the elderly (David *et al.* 1983; Nyquist & Hawthorn 1987). This is probably because the skin becomes thinner and less elastic with age. Although there were more patients over the age of 65 years with pressure sores in the 1989 survey than the 1993 survey, age is likely to continue to be a factor in tissue breakdown.

In both surveys a number of patients with pressure sores were below average weight. Although tissue wasting may be found with some diseases, it is mostly associated with poor nutrition. Malnutrition has been associated with pressure sore development (Pinchcofsky-Devin & Kaminski 1986; Cullum & Clark 1992). This is particularly important in the light of a report from the Kings Fund Centre (1992) which suggested that 50% of medical and surgical patients are malnourished.

Major surgery was the commonest factor in tissue breakdown for the 1993 survey, affecting 64.3% of patients and 40% in the 1989 survey. This finding is supported by other studies (Hicks 1971; Stotts 1988; Kemp *et al.* 1990). Bridel (1992) commented that there is still a lack of understanding of the precise factors involved in pressure sore development in the perioperative period.

For the purposes of this discussion only the numbers of patients who were bed-or chair-bound were counted in the results. However, others had some degree of reduced mobility. Reduced mobility is another factor highlighted by several studies (David *et al.* 1983; Clark *et al.* 1978; Nyquist & Hawthorn 1987). Neurological deficit has not been specifically mentioned in other studies, but many patients falling into this category also had reduced mobility.

Many other studies used the Norton score and so factors such as tissue malnutrition were not considered. As a result, it is more difficult to make comparisons with other surveys. When considering the patient population in the hospital and the particular specialities provided it can be seen that there are many acutely ill patients who are often poorly perfused undergoing extensive surgery or other types of treatment. The findings of this study confirm the vulnerability of these patients.

Assessment of some of the specific factors found in those patients with pressure sores can help to target preventive measures more effectively. They can also provide a focus for further research.

Conclusions and recommendations

After analysis of the findings of this study several conclusions and recommendations can be made.

(1) The 1993 survey shows no real reduction in the prevalence of pressure sores. This may be mainly due to increased workload.
(2) There is a reduction in the actual number of pressure sores.
(3) There is an improvement in the management of established pressure sores.
(4) More support systems are available within the hospital, but there are still inadequate numbers.
(5) Patient assessment should include assessment of nutritional status.
(6) As the patient population is stable with respect to pressure sore risk this will continue to provide the basis for planning the purchase of support systems.
(7) Education programmes are urgently needed to improve the selection and the use of support systems related to the degree of risk of the patient.
(8) Further research is necessary to identify possible causes of pressure sores within the hospital, especially within the perioperative period.
(9) Establishment of the measurement of pressure sore incidence will assist in monitoring the situation and indicate the efficacy of the prevention programme.

As National Health Service purchasing authorities continue to request information about pressure sores there will be an increasing interest in both monitoring and preventing these painful sores.

References

Anthony, D. (1989) The pressure sore debate. *Nursing Times*, **85**(26), 74.
Audit Commission (1991) *The Virtue of Patients: Making the Best Use of Ward Nursing Resources*. The Audit Commission for Local Authorities and the National Health Service in England and Wales, London.
Bliss, M.R. (1988) Prevention and management of pressure sores. *Update*, 1 May, **36**, 2258–67.
Bridel, J. (1992) Pressure sores and intra-operative risk. *Nursing Standard*, **7**(5), 28–30.

Clark, O., Barbanel, J.C., Jordan, M.M. & Nicol, M. (1978) Pressure sores. *Nursing Times,* **74**(9), 363–6.

Clark, M. & Cullum, N. (1992) Matching patient need for pressure sore prevention with the supply of pressure redistributing mattresses. *Journal of Advanced Nursing,* **17**, 310–16.

Cullum, N. & Clark, M. (1992) Intrinsic factors associated with pressure sores in elderly people. *Journal of Advanced Nursing,* **17**, 427–31.

David, J.A., Chapman, R.G., Chapman, E.J. & Lockett, B. (1983) An investigation of the current methods used in nursing for the care of patients with established pressure sores. Nursing Practice Research Unit, Northwick Park, Middlesex.

Dealey, C. (1989) The pressure sore debate. *Nursing Times,* **85**(26), 75.

Dealey, C. (1991) The size of the pressure sore problem in a teaching hospital. *Journal of Advanced Nursing,* **16**, 663–70.

Dealey, C. (1992a) Pressure sores – the result of bad nursing? *British Journal of Nursing,* **1**(15), 748.

Dealey, C. (1992b) Specific hospital problems in the prevention and management of pressure sores. *Journal of Tissue Viability,* **2**(4), 135–6.

Department of Health (1992) *Health of the Nation.* HMSO, London.

Ek, A.-C. & Boman, G. (1982) A descriptive study of pressure sores: the prevalence of pressure sores and the characteristics of patients. *Journal of Advanced Nursing,* **7**, 51–7.

Hibbs, P. (1988a) *Pressure Sore Prevention for the City and Hackney Health Authority.* City and Hackney Health Authority, London.

Hibbs, P. (1988b) Action against pressure sores. *Nursing Times,* **84**(13), 68–73.

Hicks, D.J. (1971) An incidence study of pressure sores following surgery. In *ANA Clinical Sessions: 1970 Miami,* pp. 49–54. Appleton-Century-Crofts, New York.

Ibbotson, K.A. (1988) Survey to identify the occurrence of pressure sores: preventative measures and treatments in use at Christchurch Hospital. *Care – Science and Practice,* **6**(4), 103–104.

Isaacs, S. & Michael, W.B. (1981) *Handbook in Research and Evaluation.* Edits, San Diego.

Johnson, A. (1985) A blueprint for the prevention and management of pressure sores. *Care – Science and Practice,* **2**(8), 13.

Kemp, M.G., Keithley, J.K., Smith, D.W. & Morreale, B. (1990) Factors that contribute to pressure sores in surgical patients. *Research in Nursing and Health,* **13**, 293–301.

Kings Fund Centre (1992) *A Positive Approach to Nutrition as Treatment.* Kings Fund Centre, London.

Lancet (1973) Editorial. *Lancet,* **ii**, 309.

Ling, T. & Vincent, N. (1989) Survey of pressure sores carried out on a trauma ward. *Senior Nurse,* **9**(6), 4–5.

Livesley, B. & Simpson, G. (1989) Hard cost of soft sores. *Health Service Journal,* **99**(5138), 231.

Livesley, B. & Simpson, G. (1993) *Prevention and Management of Pressure Sores within Hospital and Community Settings.* Research for Ageing Trust, London.

Lockett, B. (1983) *Prevalence and incidence in pressure sore disease.* Presented at Symposium at Royal Hospital and Home for Incurables, London.

Meehan, M. (1992) Multisite pressure ulcer prevalence survey. In *Proceedings of the 1st European Conference on Advances in Wound Management.* (Eds K.G. Harding, D. Leaper & T.D. Turner) Macmillan Magazines, London.

National Health Service Executive (1995) National Clinical Guidelines on Pressure Sore Management and Prevention. DoH, London.

Norton, D., McLaren, R. & Exton-Smith, A.N. (1975) *An Investigation of Geriatic Nursing Problems in Hospital.* Churchill Livingstone, Edinburgh.

Nyquist, R. & Hawthorn, P.J. (1987) The prevalence of pressure sores in an area health authority. *Journal of Advanced Nursing,* **12**, 183–7.

O'Dea, K. (1993) Prevalence of pressure damage in hospital patients in the UK. *Journal of Wound Care,* **2**(4), 221–5.

Panel for the Prediction and Prevention of Pressure Ulcers in Adults (1992) *Pressure Ulcers in Adults: Prediction and Prevention.* AHCPR Publication, US Department of Health and Human Services, Rockville, Maryland.

Pinchcofsky-Devin, G. & Kaminski, M.V. (1986) Correlation of pressure sores and nutritional status. *Journal of the American Geriatric Society*, **34**, 435–40.

Royal College of Nursing (1993) Survey shows hidden cuts. *Nursing Standard*, **7**(35), 23–4.

Royal College of Physicians (1986) Physical disability in 1986 and beyond. A report of the Royal College of Physicians. *Journal of the Royal College of Physicians of London*, **20**(3), 160–94.

Stotts, N.A. (1988) Predicting pressure ulcer development in surgical patients. *Heart and Lung*, **17**, 641–7.

Warner, U. & Hall, D.J. (1986) Pressure sores: a policy for prevention. *Nursing Times*, **82**(16), 59–61.

Waterlow, J. (1985) A risk assessment card. *Nursing Times*, **81**(48), 49–55.

Waterlow, J. (1988) Prevention is cheaper than cure. *Nursing Times*, **84**(25), 69–70.

Young, J. (1992) The use of specialised beds and mattresses. *Journal of Tissue Viability*, **2**(3), 79–81.

Chapter 4
The characteristics and management of patients with recurrent blockage of long-term urinary catheters

KATHRYN A. GETLIFFE, *PhD, MSc, BSc, RGN, DN Certificate*
Lecturer in Community Nursing, Department of Nursing and Midwifery, University of Surrey, Guildford, England

Encrustation and the subsequent blockage of indwelling urinary catheters is a common problem affecting up to 50% of long-term catheterized patients. For community patients, the resultant urinary bypassing or painful retention is particularly distressing since professional help is not immediately available. Catheter blockage also places increased demands on nursing time and resources. A prospective longitudinal study of 47 community patients with long-term catheters was conducted. Demographic, dietary and catheter-care data were collected, and biochemical and microbiological urinalysis conducted. Catheters were changed on three occasions, after six-week intervals, and the extent of encrustation examined. The results indicated that patients can be classified as 'blockers' and 'non-blockers'. 'Blockers' produced two or more blocked catheters and were characterized by high urinary pH and ammonium concentration. 'Blocker status' was also significantly associated with female sex and with poor mobility, but not with fluid intake and urinary output. 'Blockers' were generally managed by 'crisis care' in response to leakage or retention, rather than by planned recatheterizations prior to catheter blockage. Recognition of individual patients as 'blockers' and the establishment of a 'pattern of catheter life' would be useful to planning individualized care.

Introduction

Long-term urinary catheterization offers a practical strategy for the management of urinary dysfunction for many patients for whom alternative non-invasive methods are inappropriate or ineffective. Such patients form approximately 4% of the community nursing caseload (Roe 1987; Getliffe 1990) and may include up to 28% of patients in chronic care facilities (Kunin *et al.* 1987; Ouslander *et al.* 1987). Since a large proportion of catheterized patients are elderly, these percentages may increase as the number of elderly people in the population rises (Meredith Davies 1991).

Recurrent catheter blockage, leading to leakage of urine or painful retention, is a problem for around 50% of patients (Roe & Brocklehurst 1987; Kunin 1989), and is particularly distressing for community patients and carers, since help is not immediately available. Blockage also places increased demands on nursing time and resources, necessitating unscheduled visits, and replacement of expensive catheters. In addition, male patients may be referred to hospital for catheter changes if community nurses are untrained in male recatheterization (Kohler-Ockmore 1992).

Whilst catheter blockage is sometimes caused by bladder spasm, twisted tubing or constipation, the commonest cause is the occlusion of the lumen by hard mineral deposits or encrustations, precipitated from the urine. Encrustations may also form on the external surface of the catheter, causing pain and urethral trauma during catheter removal. The principal components of encrustations are struvite (magnesium ammonium phosphate) and calcium phosphate (Brice *et al.* 1974; Cox *et al.* 1987). These minerals precipitate from the urine under alkaline conditions produced during urinary infection with urease-producing micro-organisms, which release ammonia from urea (Griffith *et al.* 1976).

To date, management of recurrent catheter encrustation has depended largely on the use of bladder washouts to dissolve or flush out mineral deposits, or on replacement of the catheter. However, there is little research-based evidence to assist the development of effective strategies of care.

Research study

The research presented here was a comparative study of the characteristics and usual catheter management of a cohort of community patients, and formed part of a larger study which addressed the problem of catheter encrustation from both a patient-care perspective and a clinical-science perspective.

Objectives

The objectives of this part of the study were:

(1) To determine if the occurrence of catheter encrustation is a continuum experienced to some degree by all catheterized patients – or whether patients can be classified into one of two discrete groups: 'blockers' or 'non-blockers' (Kunin *et al.* 1987).
(2) To determine the factors which contribute to recurrent encrustation and blockage.

Early identification of patients as 'blockers' would assist in the planning of proactive care in contrast to reliance on reactive care when blockage occurs.

Methodology

Study population

Previous clinical studies of catheter blockage in long-term catheterized populations have been based on hospitalized patients where possible population biases such as uniformity of diet, limited mobility and the potential for cross-infection exist (Hedelin *et al.* 1985; Kunin *et al.* 1987; Mobley & Warren 1987). In this study, the population was drawn from patients living at home or in warden-controlled housing, thus minimizing these biases. Patients, resident in three district health authorities (DHA), who were expected to remain catheterized for at least four months were eligible for inclusion, providing that continuing care would be maintained by district nurses. Patients were not eligible if they were less than 16 years old, were being treated by long-term antibiotic therapy or were severely mentally confused.

It was not feasible to select a random sample since the limited target population of long-term catheterized patients in the community, and the severe disability and/or advanced age and frailty of many of those patients, restricted the numbers available. A preliminary selection was also operated by district nurses and general practitioners who excluded those patients whose medical and/or social history rendered them unsuitable for enrolment. The extent of sampling bias was limited by approaching all patients who were identified by the district nursing services within the three DHAs. Less than 8% of patients who were asked to take part in the study were unwilling to do so.

'Blockers' and 'non-blockers'

The classification of patients as 'blockers' and 'non-blockers' was dependent upon analysis of clinical specimens. Bladder washouts were withheld during the period of the study. Three used catheters, replaced at six-week intervals or earlier if the catheter became blocked, were collected from each patient. The extent of encrustation was observed by cutting the catheter open longitudinally and assigning a score of 0–4 to each 20 mm section. Observations were made by one observer to avoid inter-observer bias. Reliability was tested by the test–retest method. Ten catheters were reassessed blind after a minimum period of 10 days. This procedure was repeated on three different occasions using different groups of catheters.

Definitions

A 'blocked catheter' was defined as having at least one score of $+3$ or $+4$ where:

$+4$ = catheter lumen completely occluded
$+3$ = narrow patent channel
$+2$ = wide patent channel
$+1$ = rough surface
0 = no visible encrustation

Patients were defined as 'blockers' if two or more of their catheters became blocked during the study.

Data collection

Data relating to patient characteristics and usual catheter management were collected during semi-structured interviews with patients. Blood pressure and mobility were both measured since they may affect urinary composition, and calcium excretion in particular (Watson & Royle 1987; Cappucio *et al.* 1990). Blood pressure was measured, using an anaeroid sphygmomanometer, on two separate occasions by taking two readings five minutes apart and discarding the first reading. Patient mobility was assessed on a scale of 1–4, by discussion and, where appropriate, by observation of the patient walking from one room to another:

(1) Bed/chair-bound.
(2) Walks with an aid.
(3) Walks unaided at home only.
(4) Fully mobile.

Dietary analysis and urinary composition

Dietary intake was determined by a four-day, weighed dietary record (Fellstrom *et al.* 1989), undertaken during two weekdays and two weekend days. Dietary analysis (Table 4.1) was carried out using 'Superdiet' software (University of Surrey) in conjunction with food tables (Holland 1988, 1989, 1991; McCance 1991). Twenty-four-hour urine samples, collected during the period of the dietary study, to allow comparisons between dietary intake and urinary output compositions, were analysed for calcium, magnesium, phosphate, oxalate, urate, ammonia, citrate and protein concentrations. These components have been identified in encrusting material (Hedelin *et al.* 1984; Cox *et al.* 1987). Urinary creatinine concentrations were measured to screen for abnormal renal function.

Table 4.1 Dietary components analysed.

Fluid volume	Vitamin A	Riboflavin	Calcium	Copper
Energy	Vitamin B_6	Thiamine	Magnesium	Zinc
Protein	Vitamin B_{12}	Niacin	Sodium	Phosphate
Carbohydrate	Vitamin C	Folate	Potassium	Chloride
Fat	Vitamin D	Iron	Iodide	
Cholesterol			Selenium	
Fibre				

Pilot study

A pilot study, to test the questionnaire and interview technique, was carried out on five patients and a number of revisions to the method of coding information were made. Initial attempts to employ an analogue scale for measurement of perceived pain were abandoned when it became clear that a large number of patients had little or no sensation in the peri-urethral region.

Results

Patient characteristics

Forty-seven patients were enrolled, over 20 months. The data analysis was based on information collected from 42 patients (Table 4.2), who provided a minimum of two catheter samples. Patients excluded were: two who did not provide catheters, and three who provided only one. More patients were catheterized for incontinence 31/42; 73.8%) than for recurrent retention of urine (10/42; 23.8%) ($\chi^2 = 21.01$; $P < 0.0001$). One patient, although not incontinent, was catheterized to provide relief from diurnal and nocturnal urinary frequency.

The reliability of the observational method of assessing the quantity of encrustation was 96.3%, with the same encrustation score being recorded

Table 4.2 Study population.

	Male	Female
Sex	18	24
Median age (years)	77.5	70.0
Range (years)	58–90	27–90
Reason for catheterization		
Incontinence	9	22
Retention	9	1
Other	0	1

during the test and retest for 607/630 catheter sections. Where scores differed on the retest it was never by more than one point on the scale, and the difference was never critical to the classification of 'blockers' and 'non-blockers'. Eighteen patients (42.9%) were classed as 'blockers'. Twenty-four patients (57.1%) were classed as 'non-blockers'.

Significantly more females (14/18; 77.8%) than males (4/18; 22.2%) were 'blockers' ($\chi^2 = 4.10$; $P = 0.043$). Catheterization for incontinence was significantly correlated with being a 'blocker' (Fisher's exact test, $P = 0.028$). However, more females (22/24; 91.7%) were catheterized for incontinence than males (9/18; 50%) (Fisher's exact test, $P = 0.001$) and therefore it is unclear whether incontinence and female sex were independently related to 'blocker' status. 'Blockers' were significantly less mobile than 'non-blockers' (Mann-Whitney $U = 141.5$; $P = 0.04$) (Fig. 4.1).

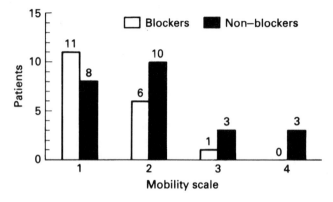

Fig. 4.1 Patient mobility.

None of the remaining items investigated (age, medical condition, blood pressure, medication, alcohol consumption, bowel habits or smoking) were correlated with 'blocker' status.

Usual catheter management

Two patients used supra-pubic catheters, and one was managed with a supra-pubic and a urethral catheter (to reduce concurrent urethral leakage of urine). Five of 15 (33.3%) patients who used hydrogel-coated catheters and 12/23 (52.2%) who used silicone elastomer-coated catheters were 'blockers', but these differences were not statistically significant. Catheter size ranged from 12 to 22 Charrière, with 50% of patients using size 14, but there was no relationship between 'blocker' status and Charrière size.

The majority of patients 32/42 (76.2%) experienced at least one recurrent problem with their catheter (Fig. 4.2). Of these problems, both leakage and

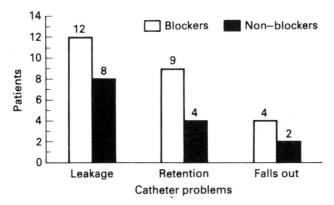

Fig. 4.2 Recurrent problems in 32/42 patients.

urinary retention were significantly associated with being a 'blocker' ($\chi^2 = 4.58$; $P = 0.032$ and $\chi^2 = 5.35$; $P = 0.021$ respectively). Four 'non-blockers' who experienced recurrent retention had 'neurogenic' bladders resulting from multiple sclerosis or spinal injury, and were subject to bladder muscle spasms.

'Blocker' status was positively correlated with the need for recatheterization in less than six weeks ($\chi^2 = 19.07$; $P = 0.0007$) (Fig. 4.3), and also with a catheter change policy of 'replacement only when the catheter becomes blocked' ($\chi^2 = 8.40$; $P = 0.0038$). By contrast, the catheters of 'non-blockers' were usually changed according to a predefined schedule. Patients had been catheterized for varying lengths of time ranging from four weeks to > 20 years, with over 45% catheterized for more than two years. Five of nine (55.6%) patients catheterized for less than six months were 'blockers', including one catheterized for just one month.

However, the length of time patients had been catheterized was not

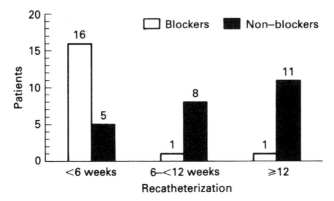

Fig. 4.3 Frequency of recatheterization prior to study.

associated with 'blocker' status, nor was the place of recatheterization, or the qualifications of the practitioner who undertook the procedure. Physical awareness of impending blockage was apparent to 13/18 'blockers' (72%). Ten of 18 (55%) felt either abdominal swelling or abdominal pain, whilst the remaining 3/18 (17%) felt slight leakage of urine only.

Use of bladder washouts

Bladder washouts were used by 15/42 (35.7%) patients prior to the commencement of the study and their regular use was significantly related to 'blocker' status (Mann-Whitney $U = 121.0$; $P = 0.0045$). All washouts were Uro-Tainer instillations (Clini-Med, High Wycombe). Suby G was the reagent used most commonly; however, the frequencies with which each reagent was used were too small to allow statistical analysis (Table 4.3).

Table 4.3   Bladder washout reagents used by 15/42 patients.

Reagent	All patients (%)	Blockers (%)	Non-blockers (%)
Chlorhexidine	7 (46.7)	5 (27.8)	2 (8.3)
Suby G	10 (66.7)	6 (33.3)	4 (16.7)
Saline	4 (26.7)	3 (16.7)	1 (4.2)
Solution R	1 (6.7)	1 (5.6)	0 (0.0)

Four patients used Suby G and chlorhexidine alternately.
Two patients used Suby G and saline alternately.
One patient used chlorhexidine and Solution R alternately.

Drainage bag care

A number of different drainage systems were in use. Nine of 42 patients (21.4%) used either a day bag or a night bag only (usually a night bag). Seventeen of 42 patients (40.5%) used a 'link system' which allowed their day bag to remain in place and a night bag to be attached to the drainage outlet, and 16/42 patients (38.1%) removed their day bag from the catheter in order to attach a night bag. None of these practices was correlated with 'blocker' status.

Care of the drainage bag varied considerably (Table 4.4). 'Blocker' status was not associated with any particular procedure. The duration of drainage-bag use varied from one to > 14 days. Ten of 42 patients (23.8%) used their bags for < 7 days, and 7/42 patients (16.7%) used them for > 14 days. The length of time for which bags were in use was not correlated with 'blocker' status, nor was there any significant relationship between patient hygiene (frequency of washing the perineal area) and being a 'blocker'.

Table 4.4 Drainage-bag care.

Care procedure	Frequency	(%)
Not re-used*	9	(21.4)
Washed with water	14	(33.3)
Washed with antiseptic	5	(11.9)
Not washed	13	(30.9)
Other†	1	(2.4)

* Not re-used: patient used one bag (day or night bag) continuously for more than 24 hours.
† Other: patient discarded both day and night bag daily.

Dietary and urinalysis

Thirty-two patients, 12 of whom were 'blockers' (37.5%), completed the four-day dietary record. Patients not participating were either elderly and infirm, or severely disabled.

Comparisons between 'blockers' and 'non-blockers' revealed no significant differences in the average daily weight (ADW) of any dietary component measured. 'Blockers' consumed more fibre than non-blockers (18.44 $\pm$ 34.17 g and 7.80 $\pm$ 3.56 g respectively), but variations within the 'blocker' group were too large to allow a significant difference to be reached. Importantly, there was no significant difference in average daily fluid intake (ADV) between 'blockers' and 'non-blockers' (ADV for 'blockers' and 'non-blockers' was 1606.6 $\pm$ 608.9 ml and 1429.1 $\pm$ 416.8 ml respectively).

Twenty-four-hour urine collections were obtained from all patients. All urinary creatinine concentrations were within the expected range for age, and for normal kidney function (males 8.8–17.0 mM/24 h; females 7.0–16.0 mM/24 h (Montgomery *et al.* 1980).

ADV was positively correlated with urinary volume (Mann–Whitney $U=0.48$; $P=0.002$) and negatively correlated with urinary magnesium and urinary phosphate (Mann–Whitney $U=-0.44$; $P=0.006$ and -0.31; $P=0.042$ respectively). High ADV was also significantly associated with greater mobility (Mann–Whitney $U=-0.32$; $P=0.035$).

Mean 24-hour urinary compositions are shown in Table 4.5. 'Blocker' status was significantly associated with high urinary pH and high urinary ammonia (two-tailed Mann–Whitney $U=63.5$; $P<0.0001$ and 112.0; $P=0.0082$ respectively), but not with urinary volume, osmolality or any other urinary component.

Table 4.5 Mean 24-hour urinary composition for 'blockers' and 'non-blockers'.

Component	Blockers	Non-blockers
	Mean ± SD	Mean ± SD
Volume	1728 ± 549.1	1549 ± 670.9
Osmolality	277.5 ± 165.6	310.5 ± 125.4
pH	7.39 ± 1.07	6.11 ± 0.665
Calcium	2.47 ± 1.64	2.19 ± 1.58
Magnesium	1.84 ± 1.54	1.91 ± 0.867
Phosphate	9.75 ± 4.36	11.8 ± 6.72
Oxalate	189.4 ± 84.4	160.5 ± 75.4
Urate	0.867 ± 0.516	1.31 ± 0.905
Ammonia	67.9 ± 76.42	23.26 ± 19.89
Citrate	0.747 ± 1.13	0.991 ± 1.17
Creatinine	4.22 ± 2.42	5.17 ± 3.05
Protein	0.201 ± 0.168	0.24 ± 0.905

Units: volume, ml; osmolality, mosmol/L; protein, g/L; oxalate, μmol/L; all other components, mM/L.

Discussion

Patient characteristics

Almost 43% of patients suffered from recurrent catheter encrustation and were classed as 'blockers'. Although no particular underlying medical condition was associated with 'blocker' status, the diseases suffered by patients indicated a high level of disability within the sample population. Less than 36% of patients were self-caring, and whilst the views of carers were not sought in this study recurrent catheter blockage undoubtedly adds to the burden of care.

Significantly more females (77.8%) than males were classed as 'blockers'. This has not been reported previously, but the majority of investigations have been restricted to patients who were predominantly of one sex (Kunin *et al.* 1987; Ouslander *et al.* 1987; Kunin 1989). However, females may be at greater risk of catheter-associated infection than males (Kunin 1987; Kennedy *et al.* 1983) since micro-organisms responsible for bacteriuria in catheterized patients are frequently present in the patient's own bowel flora (MacLaren & Peerblooms 1986), and the shorter female urethra may allow more rapid colonization.

Although a high level of disability existed amongst the whole sample population, 'blockers' were significantly less mobile than 'non-blockers' ($P < 0.05$). Kennedy *et al.* (1983) also reported that lack of mobility in community patients was a significant factor related to 'catheter problems', which included blockage, leakage and offensive smell. Such patients may be alone for long periods, with limited access to drinks and unable to alter their position to improve urinary flow.

Greater mobility might be expected to enhance unimpeded urine flow, increasing the potential for flushing out precipitated salts as they form. However, there was no correspondingly significant relationship between 'non-blockers' and high average daily fluid intake, high 24-hour urinary volume or administration of diuretic medication, all variables which would also be expected to produce increased urinary flow. Therefore, the advice commonly given to catheterized patients to 'drink plenty' to reduce mineral precipitation is not supported by this study.

Catheter management: recurrent problems and 'crisis care'

At least 76% of all patients experienced one or more recurrent problems associated with catheterization, with almost half (47%) complaining of urinary leakage, and nearly a third (32%) suffering from retention. Whilst both leakage and urinary retention were significantly associated with being a 'blocker', clearly catheterization is rarely trouble-free and nurses have an important role, not only in providing care which minimizes problems but also in educating patients and carers in catheter care, and in providing on-going support.

A prevailing tendency towards 'crisis care' existed for patients classed as 'blockers', as indicated by the practice of replacing the catheter 'only when it blocks'. Although there may be some merit in not interfering whilst the catheter is still patent, this policy fails to meet the needs of patients who urgently require help when the catheter suddenly becomes blocked. 'Blockers' had a significantly shorter time between recatheterizations than 'non-blockers' ($P < 0.0001$), with 89% of 'blockers' usually recatheterized in less than six weeks, compared to 21% of 'non-blockers'. Although the length of time catheters remained *in situ* prior to removal for blockage was variable, not only between patients who were 'blockers', but also between catheter episodes for the same patient, in over 60% of 'blockers' a pattern was identifiable.

Continued records of catheter-change frequencies may have elucidated clearer individual patterns and Norberg *et al.* (1983) have recommended monitoring three to five catheter episodes to identify a characteristic pattern of 'catheter life'. Clearly, if a pattern can be recognized, recatheterization can be planned to precede the predicted development of blockage, thus reducing the distress suffered when blockage occurs.

A policy of planned recatheterization would also reduce the pressures on community and hospital services when urgent unscheduled visits are required, or patients are sent to hospital out-patient/emergency departments for catheter changes. The majority of 'blockers' (72%) experienced early

Name: ....   District nurse: ....

                                                    Tel:...

                                                    GP: ....

                                                    Tel:...

1st assessment date: ....   2nd assessment date:..

Reason for catheterization   *History of blockage/leakage*

	Assessment 1	Assessment 2
None		
Occasional (not every catheter)		
Frequent (every catheter)		

Incontinence / Retention / Other □

Previous history of bladder calculi ....

Mobility at home

	Assessment 1	2
Bed/chair bound		
Walks with an aid		
Fully mobile		

Bladder washouts

	Assessment 1	2
None		
Reagent		
Frequency		

Catheter material

	Assessment 1	2
Hydrogel		
Silicone-elastomer		
Other		

Drainage system

	Assessment 1	2
Closed		
Link		
Valve/other		

Equipment details (to assist re-ordering):

This form may be used to aid the recognition of a characteristic pattern of 'catheter life' for patients suffering from recurrent catheter encrustation and blockage.

Fig. 4.4 Indwelling catheter assessment – establishing a pattern for planned care (side 1).

Date of catheter change	Reason for change planned/ blocked	No. days catheter in place	Urine pH	Encrustation visable?	BWO reagent and frequency	Next planned recatheterization date	Anti-biotics given?

Evaluate care plan (after three catheter 'lives')
e.g. recatheterization schedule/BWO schedule:

Evaluate care plan:

Fig. 4.4 (cont.)   Indwelling catheter assessment – establishing a pattern for planned care (side 2)

warning symptoms of impending blockage such as abdominal discomfort. Where possible, a defined course of action should be planned with nursing staff and initiated by the patient when those symptoms occur. A sample chart which may be used to help identify patients' pattern of catheter life and develop an individualized plan of management is presented in Fig. 4.4. Side 1 of the chart provides an opportunity to record patient and management characteristics which may be related to the recurrence of catheter blockage. Side 2 is designed to provide details of three 'catheter lives', including management strategies which may influence the occurrence of catheter encrustations e.g. bladder washouts, use of antibiotics (not necessarily for urinary tract infection). Measurement of urinary pH is helpful as encrustation is most likely to occur in alkaline urine. After three 'catheter lives' an attempt to recognize any pattern of blockage should be made and future catheter changes scheduled to take place prior to the likely event of blockage. The chart allows for two assessments and further charts would be required for on-going assessment and evaluation.

Reducing the risks of infection

Catheter-care practices directed towards reducing the risk of infection, e.g. drainage-bag care and personal hygiene, were unrelated to 'blocker' status despite a recognized association between encrustation and infection with urease-producers (Mobley & Warren 1987; Kunin 1989; Hedelin *et al.* 1991). Long-term catheterized patients are subject to chronic urinary infection, and micro-organisms colonizing the catheter surface as a biofilm (Nickel *et al.* 1985) provide a constant source of infection regardless of the frequency of bag changes or personal hygiene. Biofilm organisms are extremely difficult, if not impossible, to remove (Brown *et al.* 1988) and micro-organisms growing as a biofilm on the surface of drainage bags are unlikely to be eradicated by any method of cleaning the bag. Nevertheless, infecting species fluctuate over time (Breitenbucher 1984) and patients are at risk of cross-infection from carers. Therefore, it is important that clean catheter care procedures are performed by patients and aseptic procedures carried out by carers to reduce the risk of infection by potential pathogens.

Bladder washouts and catheter material

The percentage of patients using regular bladder washouts prior to the commencement of the study (36%) was lower than observed during the preliminary study (54%) (Getliffe 1990) and 44% quoted by Roe (1990). The decision to use bladder washouts and the choice of reagent is usually the responsibility of the district nurse.

The reduction in their use may be in response to recent publications highlighting potentially detrimental effects on the bladder mucosa (Elliott *et al.* 1989; Kennedy *et al.* 1992), and the resistance of catheter-associated infections to chlorhexidine (Stickler *et al.* 1987). However, the present dearth of research to support or refute the value of bladder washout procedures to diminish encrustation results in a potential imbalance of information available to nurses. An evaluation of bladder washouts using a model of the catheterized bladder was undertaken as a separate section of the main research study and is reported elsewhere (Getliffe 1994).

Suby G. which is recommended by the manufacturers to reduce encrustation, was the reagent most commonly used (60% of patients using washouts). However, the use of Suby G by 17% of all 'non-blockers' was clearly inappropriate and unnecessary. Furthermore, chlorhexidine was used by 47% of patients using washouts, despite published reports of ineffectiveness against catheter-associated infection (Stickler *et al.* 1987). Although the frequencies with which each reagent was used were too small for statistical analysis, these results suggest that some nurses are still unclear about which, if any, bladder washout is appropriate for a particular patient.

Dietary and urinary analysis

Detailed analysis of patients' diets and 24-hour urinary composition revealed that 'blockers' were characterized by high urinary pH and ammonia concentrations compared to 'non-blockers', as previously reported by others (Kunin *et al.* 1987; Kunin 1989). High ammonia concentrations and alkaline conditions are produced when urea is catalytically decomposed by urease, synthesized by infecting microorganisms. No further relationships between 'blockers' and dietary or urinary components were detected; however, wide variations in both intake and output may mask more subtle differences which exist on an individual level. Although not statistically significant, 'blockers' consumed more fibre than 'non-blockers'. This practice may have been encouraged by nurses and general practitioners, to avoid constipation as a possible cause of catheter blockage.

Conclusion

Earlier studies reported that patients with blocked catheters excreted more calcium, protein and mucin than patients whose catheters did not block (Kunin *et al.* 1987). Such results were not confirmed in the present study. Therefore, in agreement with Bruce *et al.* (1974), this study does not support the concept of a metabolic difference between 'blockers' and 'non-blockers'.

Individualized programme

Monitoring the progress and care of all patients is fundamental to nursing practice, and an individualized programme should form the focus of catheter management. However, the classification of catheterized patients into broad categories of 'blockers' and 'non-blockers' is useful in identifying those who experience recurrent catheter blockage and require a care programme directed towards relief of this problem.

Acknowledgements

The author is grateful for the award of a Nursing Research Studentship from the Department of Health, England, which allowed this study to be undertaken.

References

Breitenbucher, R. (1984) Bacterial changes in the urine samples of patients with long-term indwelling catheters. *Archives of Internal Medicine*, **144**, 1585–8.

Brown, M.R.W., Allison, D.G. & Gilbert, P. (1988) Resistance of bacterial biofilms to antibiotics: a growth related effect. *Journal of Antimicrobial Chemotherapy*, **22**, 777–83.

Bruce, A.W., Sira, S.S., Clark, A.F. & Awad, S.A. (1974) The problem of catheter encrustation. *Canadian Medical Association Journal*, **111**, 238–41.

Cappuccio, F.P., Strazzulo, P. & Mancini, M. (1990) Kidney stones and hypertension: population based study of an independent clinical association. *British Medical Journal*, **300**, 1234–6.

Cox, A.J., Harries, J.E., Hukins, D.W.L., Kennedy, A.P. & Sutton, T.M. (1987) Calcium phosphate in catheter encrustation. *British Journal of Urology*, **59**, 159–63.

Elliott, T.S.J., Reid, L., Gopal Rao, G., Rigby, R.C. & Woodhouse, K. (1989) Bladder irrigation or irritation. *British Journal of Urology*, **64**, 391–4.

Fellstrom, B., Danielson, B.G., Karlstrom, B., Lithel, H., Ljunghall, S. & Vessby, B. (1989) Dietary habits in renal stone patients compared with healthy subjects. *British Journal of Urology*, **63**, 575–80.

Getliffe, K. (1990) Catheter blockage in community patients. *Nursing Standard*, **5**, 33–6.

Getliffe, K.A. (1994) The use of bladder washouts to reduce urinary catheter encrustation. *British Journal of Urology*, **73**(6), 696–700.

Griffith, D.P., Musher, D.M. & Itin, C. (1976) Urease: the primary cause of infection-induced urinary stones. *Investigative Urology*, **13**, 346–50.

Hedelin, H., Eddeland, A., Larsson, L., Pettersson, S. & Ohman, S. (1984) The composition of catheter encrustations, including the effects of allopurinol treatment. *British Journal of Urology*, **56**, 250–54.

Hedelin, H., Larsson, L., Eddeland, A. & Pettersson, S. (1985) Factors influencing the time long-term indwelling Foley catheters can be kept *in situ*. *European Urology*, **11**, 177–80.

Hedelin, H., Bratt, C.G., Eckerdal, G. & Lincoln, K. (1991) Relationship between urease-producing bacteria, urinary pH and encrustation on indwelling urinary catheters. *British Journal of Urology*, **67**, 527–31.

Holland, B. (1988) Cereal and cereal products. Third supplement to McCance and Widdowson's *The Composition of Foods*. HMSO, London.

Holland, B. (1989) Milk products and eggs. Fourth supplement to McCance and Widdowson's *The Composition of Foods*. HMSO, London.

Holland, B. (1991) Vegetables, herbs and spices. Fifth supplement to McCance and Widdowson's *The Composition of Foods*. HMSO, London.

Kennedy, A.P., Brocklehurst, J.C. & Lye, M.D.W. (1983) Factors related to the problems of long-term catheterization. *Journal of Advanced Nursing*, **8**, 207–12.

Kennedy, A.P., Brocklehurst, J.C., Robinson, J.M. & Faragher, E.B. (1992) Assessment of the use of bladder washouts/instillations in patients with long-term indwelling catheters. *British Journal of Urology*, **70**, 610–15.

Kohler-Ockmore, J. (1992) Urinary catheter complications. *Journal of District Nursing*, **10**(8), 18–20.

Kunin, C.M. (1987) Care of the urinary catheter. In *Detection, Prevention and Management of Urinary Tract Infections*, 4th edn, p. 248. Lea and Ferbiger, Philadelphia.

Kunin, C.M. (1989) Blockage of urinary catheters. The role of micro-organisms and constituents of urine on the formation of encrustations. *Journal of Clinical Epidemiology*, **42**(9), 835–42.

Kunin, C.M., Chin, Q.F. & Chambers, S. (1987) Indwelling catheters in the elderly. Relation of catheter life to formation of encrustations in patients with and without blocked catheters. *American Journal of Medicine*, **82**, 405–11.

McCance, R. (1991) *The Composition of Foods*, 5th edn (Ed. B. Holland). HMSO, London.

MacLaren, D.M. & Peerblooms, P.G.H. (1986) Urinary infections by urea-splitting micro-organisms. In *Microbial Diseases in Nephrology*, pp. 185–93. John Wiley and Sons, London.

Meredith Davies, B. (1991) In *Community Health and Social Services*, 5th edn, p. 312. Edward Arnold, Sevenoaks, Kent.

Mobley, H.L.T. & Warren, J.W. (1987) Urease positive bacteriuria and obstruction of long-term urinary catheters. *Journal of Clinical Microbiology*, **25**, 2216–17.

Montgomery, R., Dryer, R.L., Conway, T.W. & Spector, A.A. (1980) Acid-base fluid and electrolyte control. In *Biochemistry: A Case-oriented Approach*, 3rd edn, p. 165. C.V. Mosby, St. Louis.

Nickel, J.C., Gristina, A.G. & Costerton, J.W. (1985) Electron microscopic study of an infected Foley catheter. *Canadian Journal of Surgery*, **28**, 50–52.

Norberg, B., Norberg, A. & Parkhede, U. (1983) The spontaneous variation in catheter life in long stay geriatric patients with indwelling catheters. *Gerontology*, **29**, 332–5.

Ouslander, J.G., Greengold, B. & Chen, S. (1987) Complications of chronic indwelling urinary catheters among male nursing home patients; a prospective study. *Journal of Urology*, **138**, 1191–5.

Roe, B.H. (1987) Catheter care and patient teaching. Unpublished PhD thesis. University of Manchester, Manchester.

Roe, B.H. (1990) Catheter prescribing and the use of antimicrobials. *Nursing Times*, **86**, 65–8.

Roe, B.H. & Brocklehurst, J.C. (1987) Study of patients with indwelling catheters. *Journal of Advanced Nursing*, **12**, 713–18.

Stickler, D.J., Clayton, C.L. & Chawla, J.C. (1987) The resistance of urinary tract pathogens to chlorhexidine bladder washouts. *Journal of Hospital Infection*, **10**, 28–39.

Watson, R.E. & Royle, J.A. (1987) In *Watson's Medical-Surgical Nursing and Related Physiology*, 3rd edn, pp. 517, 960. Ballière Tindall, London.

Chapter 5
Measuring feeding difficulty in patients with dementia: developing a scale

ROGER WATSON, *BSc, PhD, RGN, CBiol, MIBiol*
Senior Lecturer, Department of Nursing Studies, The University of Edinburgh,
Edinburgh, Scotland

Feeding difficulty in elderly people with dementia is well documented and the need for research in this area of nursing care has
been raised by several authors. One hundred and twelve elderly
people with dementia were entered into a study of feeding difficulty.
Data were gathered by means of a questionnaire administered to the
nurses caring for the patients. The aspects of feeding difficulty which
were investigated were based on reports of relevant behaviour in the
literature and included refusal to eat, turning the head away,
refusing to open the mouth, spitting, allowing food to drop out of
the mouth and not swallowing. It was possible to arrange these
different aspects of feeding difficulty under three headings: (1)
refusal to eat, (2) spitting, and (3) inability to swallow, and to
analyse the pattern of accumulation of these feeding difficulties by
means of Guttman scale analysis. According to this analysis, the
feeding difficulties investigated form a cumulative and unidimensional pattern. The implications of this pattern and the possibilities
for further research are discussed.

Introduction

Elderly people suffering from dementia have nutritional problems (Berlinger
& Potter 1991) and also display changes in eating behaviour as the condition
progresses (Bäckström *et al.* 1987). In the advanced stages of dementia,
difficulties with feeding are common and the case for research in this area of
caring for elderly people has been advanced by several authors (Bäckström *et
al.* 1987; Fairburn & Hope 1988a, b; Norberg *et al.* 1988; Watson 1990).

A range of difficulties and behaviour related to feeding has been described
in elderly people suffering from dementia, including difficulty in moving food
from a plate to the mouth (Athlin *et al.* 1989); difficulty with swallowing
(Norberg *et al.* 1980a; Siebens *et al.* 1986; Athlin & Norberg 1987a;
Michaelsson *et al.* 1987; Sanders 1990); behaviour indicating a refusal to eat

(Norberg *et al.* 1980a; Athlin & Norberg 1987a; Michaelsson *et al.* 1987); spitting (Norberg *et al.* 1980b; Siebens *et al.* 1986; Athlin & Norberg 1987b); leaving the mouth open so that food falls out (Siebens *et al.* 1986; Michaelsson *et al.* 1987); inability to self-feed; and complete refusal to eat (Miller 1971; Åkerlund & Norberg 1985; Alford 1986; Singh *et al.* 1988; Sanders 1990).

Research into the feeding difficulty of elderly people with dementia is needed in order to help nurses to identify the problems of individual patients and to make appropriate interventions. These interventions may be aimed at helping an individual to eat in order to improve independence, dignity and nutritional status. On the other hand, there may be circumstances where feeding is inappropriate, such as in the terminal stages of dementia.

An understanding of the feeding difficulties of elderly people with dementia, gained through research, may help nurses to make decisions about interventions aimed at improving food intake at different stages of the condition.

The study

It has been argued that one of the initial requirements for research into the feeding difficulties of elderly people with dementia is a method whereby the level of difficulty with feeding, in individual patients, can be measured (Watson 1983a). It was the objective of the research reported in this chapter to develop such a method.

'Feeding' refers to the act of moving food from a plate, to the mouth, and then swallowing it, after Siebens *et al.* (1986). 'Difficulty' refers to any behaviour related to feeding which will result in a reduced intake of food.

Methods

The present study was conducted by means of a questionnaire, and the items for the questionnaire (Table 5.1) were based on the difficulties identified by the authors referred to in the introduction. Data collection took place in two 'rounds' which were separated by 6 months (November 1991 and May 1992). Factor analysis showed that all of these items loaded on one factor (following principal components analysis and oblique rotation) described as 'patient obstinacy/passivity' (Watson & Deary 1994).

Charge nurses in four wards of a psychogeriatric unit were asked to identify subjects in their care who had the diagnosis of dementia. Once the subjects had been identified the questionnaires were sent to the wards and distributed to the leaders of the nursing teams on the wards for completion.

Table 5.1 Questionnaire administered to nurses in present study.

Q1 Does the patient ever refuse to eat?
Q2 Does the patient turn his head away while being fed?
Q3 Does the patient refuse to open his mouth?
Q4 Does the patient spit out his food?
Q5 Does the patient leave his mouth open allowing food to drop out?
Q6 Does the patient refuse to swallow?

The response to the questions was either: A, never; B, sometimes; C, often.
References
Q1 (Miller 1971; Åkerlund & Norberg 1985; Alford 1986; Singh *et al.* 1988; Sanders 1990).
Q2 (Norberg *et al.* 1980a; Athlin & Norberg 1987a; Michaelsson *et al.* 1987).
Q3 (Athlin & Norberg 1987a; Michaelsson 1987).
Q4 (Norberg *et al.* 1980b; Siebens *et al.* 1986; Athlin & Norberg 1987b).
Q5 (Siebens *et al.* 1986; Michaelsson *et al.* 1987).
Q6 (Norberg *et al.* 1980a; Siebens *et al.* 1986; Michaelsson *et al.* 1987; Athlin & Norberg 1987a; Sanders 1990).

The means whereby the questionnaires were administered and completed was approved by the charge nurses.

It was felt that it would be appropriate to exploit the nursing teams used in this particular setting as this would ensure that the nurses completing the questionnaires would be familiar with the individual subjects. The expected responses to the questions were either 'never', 'sometimes' or 'often' which were indicated by answering either A, B or C respectively. For reasons described below, the responses to the questions were dichotomized to 'yes' and 'no' respectively, and these responses were denoted as 1 and 0 respectively.

Scale analysis

The results of the present study were analysed by attempting to arrange the responses to the questionnaire into a scale according to the method of Guttman (Guttman 1950), hereafter referred to as the Guttman scale. The main characteristics of such a scale are that it is both cumulative and unidimensional in nature. The score given to an individual from a Guttman scale in fact identifies which items on the scale have been ascribed to that individual.

In order to illustrate this, the example used by Williams *et al.* (1976) of a scale for recovery of a sick person will be used. It is essential that any scale has construct validity such that the scale behaves in accordance with an intuitive construct of the problems under consideration. Three activities which are obviously cumulative in nature and which measure the phenomenon of recovery are: getting up; going out of the house; going back to work.

If a score is ascribed to an individual based on the number of the above items which apply to them then, from that score, it is possible to specify which items apply to that individual. There are four possible scores from what are described as the 'scale types' for the above recovery pattern if 0 is taken to indicate that an item does not apply and 1 is taken to indicate that an item does apply to an individual who is recovering (Table 5.2). A score of 0 indicates that the person has not started to recover and a score of 3 indicates that the person is fully recovered, according to the items of the scale.

To quote Williams *et al.* (1976):

'If a group consists entirely of scale types, we can say that the cumulative scale concerned is unidimensional for that group. However, a perfect scale is improbable: measurement error, sampling error, and random variation among individuals militate against perfection.'

Table 5.2 A Guttman scale composed entirely of scale types.

Score	Scale types
3	111
2	110
1	100
0	000

Note: 0 indicates that a trait is absent; 1 indicates that a trait is present.

Non-scale types

In addition, therefore, to the above scale types there are likely, due to the reasons described above by Williams *et al.* (1976), to be non-scale types as follows: 101, 011, 001, 010. Such non-scale types will lead to errors in the scale and the methods which are used to test the existence of hypothesized scales are concerned with measuring the proportion of errors. The conventions for the use of these measures are quite stringent since they do not allow an interpretation of the scale in terms of sampling error. Moreover, it is recommended that scales are replicated to safeguard against the possibility of chance events leading to the apparent confirmation of a hypothesized scale.

Two coefficients express the levels of error at which scales are considered to be cumulative and unidimensional and these are the coefficient of reproducibility and the coefficient of scalability. The coefficient of reproducibility expresses the number of errors in a scale as a proportion of the total number of items which have been responded to and the coefficient of scalability expresses the proportion of the number of errors which could have been predicted after taking into account the extremeness of items in the scale.

The latter coefficient is an important adjunct to the coefficient of reproducibility as it is obviously quite possible to obtain a reproducible scale if all of the responses to the items in a scale for all subjects investigated is the same. Conventionally, the coefficient of reproducibility and the coefficient of scalability should be greater than 0.9 and 0.6 respectively in order to confirm the existence of a valid cumulative and unidimensional Guttman scale.

It is true to say that the statistical significance of a Guttman scale cannot be estimated in terms of sampling error – since little is known about the distribution criteria of such scales. It is possible, however, to calculate the significance of the distribution of subjects between scale and non-scale types as described by Schuessler (1961). In this method, the proportion of individuals responding to each of the items is calculated and these proportions are used to calculate the expected frequencies of the scale and non-scale types. This information, along with the observed frequencies of scale and non-scale types, is used to calculate a value of chi-square, which can be compared, at the appropriate degree of freedom, with tabulated values of chi-square. By these means it is possible to minimize the possibility of ascribing scalability to a chance distribution of responses.

Indicators of feeding difficulty

The six items from the questionnaire in Table 5.1, which were based on descriptions of feeding difficulties observed in elderly patients with dementia and reported in the literature, were arranged under three headings. These headings were indicators of feeding difficulty and, apart from being a convenient way in which to scale analyse the questionnaire, these headings were also considered to have 'construct validity' as described by Williams *et al.* (1976). The three headings, and their respective questions (Table 5.1) were:

(1) Behaviour indicating refusal to eat (questions 1, 2 and 3).
(2) Spitting (question 4).
(3) Not swallowing (questions 5 and 6).

Arranging items for scale analysis, as shown above, is a legitimate procedure since the possibility of falsely producing a scale, where none exists, is guarded against by testing for scalability as described by Menzel (1953). Where questions were combined under headings, such as heading 1 (questions 1, 2 and 3), a positive response for one or more of the questions was taken to indicate a positive response for that heading.

Trichotomous analysis

Previous analysis of the data presented in this paper has demonstrated that it is possible to obtain a reproducible and scalable pattern of responses to the questions as they were presented to the nurses in the study (Watson 1993b). This analysis involves setting up a trichotomous series of responses across the three indicators of feeding difficulty.

There are a number of disadvantages in this approach. First, while a potentially more sensitive six-point scale is produced, the clinical applicability of such a scale is doubtful compared with the four-point scale which is the outcome of the present analysis. Second, using the trichotomous analysis, the scale proved not to be replicable and this is undoubtedly due to the greater possibility for error by the nurses in differentiating between subjects who 'never', 'sometimes' or 'often' display a feeding difficulty compared with differentiating whether a feeding difficulty is either present or absent, which is the effective outcome of the dichotomous analysis. Third, the trichotomous scale does not lend itself to analysis of the statistical significance of the distribution between scale and non-scale types, as is the case with the dichotomous scale.

For the above reasons, the present data were dichotomized into responses which indicated whether or not a feeding difficulty was either present or absent. These were denoted as described above and the outcome was that the present analysis was testing for the validity, in terms of cumulation and unidimensionality of a four-point scale from 0 to 3 as shown in Table 5.3. This table also shows the questions which could be asked by nursing staff in order to evaluate feeding difficulty in individual elderly patients with dementia and thereby obtain a score according to the EdFED Scale (Edinburgh Feeding in Dementia Scale).

Table 5.3 EdFED Scale #1*. The highest number of questions for which the answer is 'Yes' indicates the position of the patient on the EdFED scale.

Score	Description	
0	No apparent feeding difficulty	
1	Behaviour indicating refusal	
2	Spitting	
3	Refusal/inability to swallow	
Questions		
1	Does the patient indicate refusal to eat e.g. turning the head away or refusing to open the mouth?	Yes/No
2	Does the patient spit food out?	Yes/No
3	Does the patient refuse or show an inability to swallow e.g. keeping food in the mouth or allowing food to drop out of the mouth?	Yes/No

* Edinburgh Feeding Evaluation in Dementia. This scale is described as #1 because it is likely to undergo subsequent modification.

Results

The study reported here was carried out in two stages. A total of 112 elderly patients with dementia were entered into the study. Seventy of these subjects were common to both stages of the study and a full breakdown of the subjects entered into the study, in terms of diagnosis (as reported by nursing staff) and survival, is given in Table 5.4.

Table 5.4 Profile of subjects in the study. The diagnoses were those which were reported by the nursing staff on the basis of the diagnoses recorded for each subject in the medical case notes. The number of subjects who died between the two parts of the study, and the concomitant survivors, are shown in brackets.

Medical diagnosis*	No.
Senile dementia	74
Senile dementia of the Alzheimer's type	28
Pre-senile dementia	7
Multi-infarct dementia	2
Korsakov's dementia	1

Entry into study and survival

Entry date	Died	Left	Survivors	Data
November 1991				
95	7	2	86	85*
	(16	—	70)	
May 1992				
17	2	4	81	81

* One spoiled data sheet.

The majority of the subjects were reported by nursing staff as having senile dementia, with the next largest group reported as specifically having Alzheimer's disease.

Ninety-five subjects were initially recruited into the study and, due to death, leaving the area in which the study was being conducted and a spoiled data collection sheet, data were collected from 85 subjects in the first part of the study (Table 5.4). Sixteen subjects died in the period between the two stages of the study and a further 17 were recruited. The death of two subjects and four leaving the area in which the study was being conducted resulted in data being collected from 81 subjects in the second stage of the study.

A summary of the results of the present study is shown in Table 5.5. It can be seen that the data from both stages of the study yield about 90% of scale types (88% in the first stage and 87% in the second stage). The results of the

Table 5.5 Guttman scale analysis of feeding difficulty.

	November 1991	June 1992
Subjects	85	81
% Scale types	88	0
C of R	0.93	0.93
C of S	0.63	0.63
χ^2 5 d.f.	36.9*	72.9*

C of R, coefficient of reproducibility.
C of S, coefficient of scalability.
*$P < 0.001$.

chi-square analysis of the distribution of the subjects between scale and non-scale types show that these are highly significant. At both stages of the study the coefficients of reproducibility and scalability (significant to two decimal places) indicate that the scale is cumulative and unidimensional. Subsequent replication of the study on another unit yielded results, not shown in this chapter, which were satisfactory in terms of reproducibility and scalability (Watson 1994a).

Discussion

The questionnaire used in this study was designed to incorporate the feeding difficulties of elderly people with dementia which have been reported in the literature. It was important, for the purposes of the study, to indicate what the expected problems of the subjects might be in order to gather data across several wards which could then be combined for the purpose of analysis.

The method of data collection depended on the clinical experience of the team leaders and on their knowledge of the individual patients in their care. It has already been demonstrated, in other studies, that valid information about the needs of patients can be obtained in this way (Schnelle & Traughber 1983; Fries & Cooney 1985). The alternative would have been to use trained data collectors who visited the wards during the study. It was felt, however, that better cooperation would be obtained, in this instance, from the wards if the clinical expertise of the nurses in the wards was used to provide data. Hopefully, this avoided the 'conflict of interest' described by le Roux (1988) which often exists between clinicians and researchers.

The results of the study indicate that it is possible to establish a pattern for the development of feeding difficulty in elderly people with dementia. There is a logical progression of difficulty, beginning with behaviour which indi-cates that the individual is beginning to refuse to eat. These problems, according to the present study, include refusing to eat, turning the head away and refusing to open the mouth. The next stage is characterized by spitting and, finally, there is an inability to swallow, either by being unable to carry this out or by allowing food to drop out of the mouth.

Implications of the present study

The majority of subjects in the present study were suffering from senile dementia. It has already been established that changes in eating, such as those described in this paper, are probably a unique feature of dementia (Fairburn & Hope 1988b) and it is known that the terminal stages of dementia are characterized by the failure of spoon-feeding (Norberg *et al.* 1980b).

It is possible, therefore, that the underlying dimension or construct in the present study, which dictates the pattern of feeding ability observed in individual patients (and thereby their position on the Guttman scale), is physical and mental deterioration due to the progression of the dementing condition.

Alternatively, the underlying dimension, which establishes the cumulative pattern of difficulty with feeding, could be the nursing intervention which the patients receive in response to their initial difficulty with feeding or refusal to eat. This latter possibility is worthy of further investigation.

Limitations of the present study

The present study was carried out on a convenience sample of elderly patients with dementia. For this reason, since the sample was not random, it is not possible to generalize the results to all elderly patients with dementia. The scale was replicated within the present study, the majority of the subjects being common to both parts of the study. This replication showed that, within the environment where the scale was developed and tested, it is replicable.

Since the tests for validity of the scale, which were applied in this work, do not measure statistical significance in terms of sampling error, it is all the more necessary to carry out replication. The sample size, however, is comparable to sample sizes used in order to establish reproducibility and scalability in other published studies (Menzel 1953).

The validity of the scale is based on the fact that the questions which were included in the questionnaire came from the literature on the problems of feeding in elderly patients with dementia. Validity, in any other sense, is hard to confirm with any measurement scale but there are ways in which an insight into the present scale could be gained by investigating its clinical significance. Preliminary studies have shown that nurses do recognise the order of stages in the Guttman scale (Watson 1994b). There are also moderate correlations between EdFED scores and several aspects of nursing care (Watson 1994a).

Conclusion

A questionnaire has been constructed whereby information about the feeding difficulty of individuals in a group of elderly people with dementia has been obtained.

The data were collected by nurses working with the individual subjects and this has proved to be a convenient and, within the constraints of the present study, reliable method of data collection.

A scoring system for the development of feeding difficulty by elderly people with dementia has been produced and the validity of this scoring system, within the constraints of the present study, has been tested by analysis of scale according to the method of Guttman (1950). Further work requires to be done in order to test the reliability of the scale in other environments.

Acknowledgements

This study was supported by funding from the Gardner Bequest to the Department of Nursing Studies at the University of Edinburgh.

References

Åkerlund, B.M. & Norberg, A. (1985) An ethical analysis of double bind conflicts as experienced by care workers feeding severely demented patients. *International Journal of Nursing Studies*, **22**, 207–16.

Alford, D.M. (1986) Behavioural responses of the institutionalized elderly to eating and to food services. *Nursing Homes*. January/February, 20–24.

Athlin, E. & Norberg, A. (1987a) Caregiver's attitudes to and interpretations of the behaviour of severely demented patients during feeding in a patient assignment care system. *International Journal of Nursing Studies*, **24**, 145–53.

Athlin, E. & Norberg, A. (1987b) Interaction between the severely demented patient and his caregiver during feeding. *Scandinavian Journal of Caring Science*, **1**, 117–23.

Athlin, E., Norberg, A., Axelsson, K., Möller, A. & Nordström, G. (1989) Aberrant eating behaviour in elderly Parkinsonian patients with and without dementia: analysis of video recorded meals. *Research in Nursing and Health*, **12**, 41–51.

Bäckström, Å., Norberg, A. & Norberg, B. (1987) Feeding difficulties in long stay patients at nursing homes. Caregiver turnover and caregiver's assessments of duration and difficulty of assisted feeding and amount of feed received by the patient. *International Journal of Nursing Studies*, **24**, 69–76.

Berlinger, W.G. & Potter, J.F. (1991) Low body mass index in demented outpatients. *Journal of the American Geriatrics Society*, **39**, 973–8.

Fairburn, C.G. & Hope, R.A. (1988a) Change in behaviour in dementia: a neglected research area. *British Journal of Psychiatry*, **152**, 406–407.

Fairburn, C.G. & Hope, R.A. (1988b) Changes in eating in dementia. *Neurobiology of Ageing*, **9**, 28–9.

Fries, B.E. & Cooney, L.M. (1985) Resource utilisation groups: a patient classification system for long-term care. *Medical Care*, **23**(2), 110–22.

Guttman, L. (1950) The basis for scalogram analysis. In *Measurement and Prediction* (Eds. S.A. Stouffer, L. Guttman, E.A. Suchman, P.F. Lazarsfeld, S.A. Star & J.A. Clausen), pp. 60–90. Princeton University Press, Princeton.

le Roux, A.A. (1988) Conflict of interest. *Nursing Times*, **84**(29), 32–3.

Menzel, H. (1953) A new coefficient for scalogram analysis. *Public Opinion Quarterly*, **17**, 268–80.

Michaelsson, E., Norberg, A. & Norberg, B. (1987) Feeding methods for demented patients in end stage of life. *Geriatric Nursing*. March/April, 69–73.

Miller, M.B. (1971) Unresolved feeding and nutrition problems of the chronically ill elderly. *The Gerontologist*, **11**, 329–36.

Norberg, A. Bäckström, Å., Athlin, E. & Norberg, B. (1988) Food refusal amongst nursing home patients as conceptualized by nurses' aids and enrolled nurses: an interview study. *Journal of Advanced Nursing*, **13**, 478–83.

Norberg, A., Norberg, B. & Bexell, G. (1980a) Ethical problems in feeding patients with advanced dementia. *British Medical Journal*, **281**, 847–9.

Norberg, A., Norberg, B., Gippert, H. & Bexell, G. (1980b) Ethical conflicts in long-term care of the aged: nutritional problems and the patient-care worker relationship. *British Medical Journal*, **280**, 377–8.

Sanders, H.N. (1990) Feeding dependent eaters among geriatric patients. *Journal of Nutrition in the Elderly*, **9**(3), 69–74.

Schnelle, J.F. & Traughber, B. (1983) A behavioural assessment system applicable to geriatric nursing facility residents. *Behavioural Assessment*, **5**, 231–43.

Schuessler, K. (1961) A note on statistical significance of scalogram. *Sociometry*, **24**, 312–18.

Siebens, H., Trupe, E., Siebens, A., Cook, F., Anshen, S., Hanauer, R. *et al.* (1986) Correlates and consequences of eating dependency in institutionalised elderly. *Journal of the American Geriatrics Society*, **34**, 192–8.

Singh, S., Mulley, G.P. & Losowsky, M.S. (1988) Why are Alzheimer patients thin? *Age and Ageing*, **17**, 21–8.

Watson, R. (1990) Feeding patients who are demented. *Nursing Standard*, **4**(44), 28–31.

Watson, R. (1993a) Measuring feeding difficulty in patients with dementia; perspectives and problems. *Journal of Advanced Nursing*, **18**, 25–31.

Watson, R. (1993b) Estimating the relative level of feeding difficulty in elderly patients with dementia. British Feeding and Drinking Group Annual Meeting. University of Sussex, Brighton, 25–26 March.

Watson, R. (1994a) Measuring feeding difficulty in patients with dementia: replication and validation of the EdFED Scale #1. *Journal of Advanced Nursing*, **19**, 850–55.

Watson, R. (1994b) Measurement of feeding difficulty in patients with dementia. *Journal of Psychiatric and Mental Health Nursing*, **1**, 45–6.

Watson, R. & Deary, I.J. (1994) Measuring feeding difficulty in patients with dementia: multivariate analysis of feeding problems, nursing interventions and indicators of feeding difficulty. *Journal of Advanced Nursing*, **20**, 283–7.

Williams, R.G.A., Johnston, M., Wallis, L.A. & Bennet, A.E. (1976) Disability: a model and measurement technique. *British Journal of Preventative and Social Medicine*, **30**, 71–8.

Chapter 6
Nurses' role in informing breast cancer patients: a comparison between patients' and nurses' opinions

TARJA SUOMINEN, RN, PhD
Assistant Professor, Department of Nursing, University of Turku, Turku, Finland

HELENA LEINO-KILPI, PhD, RN
Associate Professor, Department of Nursing, University of Turku, Turku, Finland

and PEKKA LAIPPALA, PhD
Associate Professor, Department of Public Health/Biometry Unit, University of Tampere, Tampere, Finland

A study was conducted to determine which nursing care activities in informing breast cancer patients are considered important by the patients themselves and their nurses. One hundred and nine breast-operated women and 125 nurses participated in the study. All patients had contracted breast cancer in the previous three years but not within the previous three months. Ward and clinical nurses from one university and six area hospitals were contacted. The patients considered that the information that they had received and their level of knowledge of their own situation was not conducive to good recovery. The nurses' opinions were in agreement, although their overall assessment of the situation was more positive.

Introduction

It is estimated that the incidence of breast cancer will be 3700 by the year 2006 in Finland (Hakulinen *et al.* 1989) where the total population numbers about five million. Breast cancer has been the most common malignant disease among Finnish women since the 1960s (Pukkala *et al.* 1987). However, most breast cancer patients are actively engaged in working life and their possibilities of recovery and rehabilitation are good. The care provided by health care workers for women with breast cancer should be as effective as possible, because it supports good recovery in so many women.

The research carried out on the care of patients with breast cancer is important for every society from the humanitarian and economic point of view. The purpose of this study was to investigate how breast-operated cancer patients and their nurses assessed the information that patients received before, during and after hospitalization and to evaluate what role the nurses caring for cancer patients had in providing information.

Literature review

Being ill with cancer is stressful both for the patients and their relatives (Oberst & James 1985; Northouse & Swain 1987; Aaronson *et al.* 1988). Cancer of the breast has been shown to have psychological and social effects on patients (Lindsey *et al.* 1981; Hailey *et al.* 1988; Cawley *et al.* 1990; Graydon 1994; Schain *et al.* 1994; Willits 1994). As with any long-term illness, information becomes crucial for patients, enabling them to devise realistic expectations in self-care, adapting to lifestyle changes and coping with the diagnosis (Cassileth *et al.* 1980; Fredette 1990).

It is obvious that most patients prefer to be well informed about their situation (Lazarus & Folkman 1984; Mishel 1984; Dodd 1988; Bubela *et al.* 1990) because they use cognitive mediation to cope with stressful events (Padilla *et al.* 1981; Hartfield *et al.* 1982; Ziemer 1983; Sime & Libera 1985). However, individuals differ in their receptiveness to information and readiness for self-care in treatment situations (Krantz *et al.* 1980). During the illness experience women seek information about their cancer treatment and related physical care. The importance of assessing the breast cancer patients' received informational needs at various points is obvious in the treatment continuum (Harrison-Woermke & Graydon 1993).

Many patients with cancer live with uncertainties (Plant *et al.* 1987) and insufficient information about their illness (see for example, Derdiarian 1986; Fredette & Beattie 1986). In this connection uncertainty is operationally defined, not as an emotion, but as a lack of illness-related knowledge (Molleman *et al.* 1984). Patients do not have sufficient illness-related knowledge to participate in making treatment decisions (Mackillop *et al.* 1988). However, many studies have found that it is female, single and well-educated patients that primarily want to have an active role in decision-making (Cassileth *et al.* 1980; Givio 1986; Blanchard *et al.* (1988).

Larson (1984) carried out a study to determine which nursing care activities are considered most important by patients and found that patients with cancer rank information highly and consider the trusting relationship sub-scale to be least important. Comstock *et al.* (1982) reported that patient satisfaction is only weakly correlated with empathy. Bartlett *et al.* (1984) obtained contradictory results showing that the quality of interpersonal skills has a greater influence on satisfaction than the quantity of patient education.

Information needs

Little is known about how patients with breast cancer perceive their informational needs and how they assess the information that they have received. Ward & Griffin (1990) suggested that breast cancer patients' informational needs are not adequately met. However, it is not clear whether this deficit is present because clinicians do not provide sufficient information, or because patients do not absorb information or whether it is due to an interaction of these two factors.

Although some studies have been carried out on patient information from both the patients' and the physicians' viewpoint (Pfefferbaum & Levenson 1982), and shown communication problems with the medical team (Lerman *et al.* 1993), the role of nurses in information delivery has received little attention.

According to Leino-Kilpi (1990) the nurse is the dominant party in the information process. Certain elements in the nurse's activity support patients in their efforts to cope independently; guidance, education, motivation and even indoctrination. Guidance and motivation may be related to present or future activities (Close 1988; Wilson-Barnett 1988; Neufeld *et al.* 1993; Hack *et al.* 1994). These activities are carried out by nurses who have the necessary knowledge and/or skills (Leino-Kilpi 1990).

Tilley *et al.* (1987) showed that incongruities occurred between nurses' and patients' perceptions of the nurse's role in patient education. However, the nursing intervention may improve women's sense of control, and further changes in care are needed to meet their psychosocial needs, such as adequate information about medical treatment and more 'conforming' relationships (Pålsson & Norberg 1995). Although patients identified a general teaching function for nurses, they preferred to receive the specific information related to their condition from a physician. Patients do not always identify nurses as teachers, but nurses usually seem to consider nurses themselves as competent and preferable patient educators (Pender 1974; Summers 1984). However, there are several obstacles to patient education by nurses. Nurses may have insufficient teaching resources, or support from other professional groups and from nursing administrators may be lacking (Wilson-Barnett & Osborne 1983).

The study

The study data were collected in the spring of 1989 from breast cancer patients who had contracted cancer in the previous three years (but not within the previous three months) and in the spring of 1990 from nurses caring for breast cancer patients in south-western Finland.

Samples

The random sample consisted of 140 Finnish women who had been operated on for breast cancer. One hundred and nine patients (N1), 78% of the sample, responded to the questionnaire. The patients were aged between 32 and 78 years. Most women had undergone radical mastectomies, and some had also received other treatments. In 44% of the women, the time between detection of cancer and initiation of this study was less than one year.

The sample of nurses consisted of 176 radiological and registered ward and clinical nurses who mainly cared for breast cancer patients in one university and six area hospitals. One hundred and twenty-five nurses (N2), 71% of the sample, returned the questionnaire. Eighty-nine nurses were from wards and 36 nurses from clinics. Surgical wards accounted for 62% of them and radiological wards for 12%. Clinical nurses accounted for 26% of the sample, 9% of them being radiological nurses. The average period of employment of the nurses was 15 years, and they all had considerable experience of cancer patients, with an average employment of 12 years in cancer wards and clinics.

Study tools

Two questionnaires were developed separately for nurses and patients and pre-tested on patients as well as ward and clinical nurses. The questionnaires were largely identical. The first section assessed patients' readiness and resources for participation and in the second section patients were asked to report how they perceived the information and supporting guidance that they had received. The care of breast cancer patients was carefully examined in the part of the study that focused on nurses.

Data analysis

Statistical analysis of the data was based on percentage distribution, correlations and cross-tabulations. The samples (N1 = 109 and N2 = 125) were analysed using log-linear models. The method has previously been described in greater detail by Agresti (1984, 1990).

The comparison of the two sets of data in the present study was made at content level, and statistical analysis was used as a formal tool to support the conceptual content of the comparison problem. Patients' perspective is dissimilar to that of nurses. Thus, statistical analysis of two such different groups was not considered conceptually reasonable. However, comparison of the models developed was possible at content level. It was possible to identify those issues that are important for patients and nurses as far as the breast cancer patient's knowledge of her own situation is concerned.

Results

Information obtained before and during hospitalization

Breast cancer patients' illness-related knowledge was first measured on the basis of five variables. Table 6.1 shows the results.

Table 6.1   Information received by breast cancer patients before hospitalization according to patients ($n = 109$) and nurses ($n = 125$).

Variables for patients receiving information	Level of information (%)				
	None	Little	Unknown	Considerable	Very considerable
Disease	28 (1)	50 (56)	3 (12)	15 (30)	4 (1)
Treatment	43 (5)	34 (57)	8 (12)	13 (24)	2 (2)
Operations	47 (8)	40 (51)	3 (24)	9 (15)	1 (2)
Internal prosthesis	83 (23)	8 (42)	1 (29)	6 (5)	2 (1)
External prosthesis	47 (7)	31 (46)	2 (22)	14 (23)	6 (2)

Table 6.1 indicates that nurses had much more positive views on the information received by patients before hospitalization than the patients themselves. However, nurses also reported that breast cancer patients did not receive enough information. About half of the nurses considered that patients knew very little about their disease situation, whereas nearly half of the patients thought that they knew hardly anything about their future treatments and operations.

On the other hand, only a few patients and nurses considered that breast cancer patients are sufficiently informed on admission to the hospital for treatments. Breast cancer patients' illness-related knowledge was also measured in relation to their hospitalization (Table 6.2).

Table 6.2   Information received by breast cancer patients as assessed by the patients themselves ($n = 109$) and by nurses ($n = 125$).

Issues for patients receiving information	Level of information (%)				
	None	Little	Unknown	Considerable	Very considerable
Economic support	53 (21)	21 (53)	5 (4)	17 (19)	4 (3)
Disease	12 (3)	52 (42)	4 (4)	27 (43)	5 (8)
Treatment	37 (13)	46 (40)	4 (10)	9 (33)	4 (4)
Operations	50 (35)	36 (48)	4 (5)	6 (9)	4 (3)
Internal prosthesis	79 (36)	17 (46)	1 (9)	1 (8)	2 (1)
External prosthesis	23 (15)	40 (32)	2 (5)	28 (44)	7 (4)

Table 6.2 indicates that breast cancer patients did not consider themselves well-informed about their illness situation in the hospital. Most nurses agreed on this. However, nurses reported that patients were well-informed about their disease and treatments. They also reported that they gave patients information on external prostheses.

Breast cancer patients' informational guidance

Patients and nurses were asked the same questions about the illness-related knowledge of the patients. Breast cancer patients and nurses stressed different parts of the informational area. However, all study variables measured the same content area.

The log-linear model for the patients included the following interactions (interaction marked by an asterisk):

Information received by patients about examinations*
Information received by patients about hospitalization +
Patients' knowledge level on admission to the hospital*
Information received by patients during their hospital stay +
Information received by patients about examinations*
Information received by patients during hospital stay

In the above model $G^2 = 8.72$, d.f. = 8, $P = 0.37$. Statistical analysis gives information about the goodness-of-fit of the model, where a high P-value is indicative of a satisfactory model (Agresti 1984, 1990).

For the nurses, the following interactions were found (interaction marked by an asterisk):

Patients' insufficient knowledge level during hospital stay*
Patients' knowledge level on admission +
Patient's insufficient knowledge level during hospital stay*
Information received by patients about examinations*
Information received by patients during hospital stay +
Patients' information resources before hospitalization*
Patients' insufficient knowledge level during hospital stay

In this model $G^2 = 50.37$, d.f. = 82, $P = 0.98$.

When the nurses caring for breast cancer patients assumed that the patient had received much information from various sources before hospitalization, they were also better aware of the patients' knowledge level during hospitalization.

For patients the variable 'information received about examinations' seemed to have a central position among 'information received' variables. When breast cancer patients reported that they were sufficiently informed about examinations, their knowledge about different factors involving breast cancer would increase, and they would thus have a better opportunity to formulate and ask questions. A patient's good knowledge of her own situation and the information received before hospitalization also improve the patient's possibilities of receiving information about examinations.

Hospital nurses who were aware about areas where breast cancer patients had sufficient knowledge tended to think that patients were well-informed by doctors and nurses about their own situation even before hospitalization.

Furthermore, if breast cancer patients were not informed about the purpose of examinations, they felt that they missed information during their hospitalization. When patients were informed about examinations, they also felt that they had received information about the illness itself, possible treatments and economic support available.

Nurses reported that they informed patients about single issues such as economic support and prostheses, although they were not willing to define the areas where patients had insufficient knowledge. However, most nurses reported that they explained to patients about examinations, gave information and also tried to find out what matters patients expected to receive more information about.

Discussion

The results were in many ways similar to other findings about this subject. Our statistical analysis was based on a multivariate technique and, accordingly, we could study simultaneous dependence structures in greater detail. If breast cancer patients had received information, their recovery also seemed to be better. This finding is in agreement with the results of previous studies, for example, that by Lazarus & Folkman (1984). However, if patients felt that they were not well-informed before hospitalization, they were not well-equipped to ask questions about their situation in the hospital either. The role of nurses in informing patients seemed to be important even before hospitalization. Breast cancer patients expected information both from nurses and doctors during their illness experience.

Those nurses who were interested in evaluating how much patients knew about their situation were also willing to inform their patients. Nurses should try to identify those patients who are not well-informed, because information seemed to promote recovery in cancer patients, which is in agreement with a report by Larson (1984).

Insufficient information

According to the present study, breast cancer patients were not given sufficient information and their level of knowledge of their own situation was not conducive to good recovery. Derdiarian (1986), Fredette (1990), Mackillop *et al.* (1988) and Ward & Griffin (1990) reported similar findings. Log-linear modelling made it possible to analyse data multi-dimensionally. It was even possible to study the dependence structure of three variables. One finding was that patients' low knowledge level about their situation affected almost all other aspects of their illness studied.

Thus, by informing patients adequately, the hospital staff could compensate for knowledge gaps originating from the time before hospitalization and support them on the road to recovery. However, neither patients nor nurses were clear about nurses' role in patient education. This result is in agreement with the findings of Pender (1974) and Tilley *et al.* (1987) who emphasized that nurses need to develop a clear definition of their role in patient education.

Implications for further studies

Research is needed to define what kind of information breast cancer patients prefer to receive and in what form they like to receive this information at the various stages of their illness. Organizational factors within the health care system, which encourage or discourage nurses as effective patient educators, should be investigated. Log-linear modelling is one statistical method for the investigation of multi-dimensional dependence structures in the field of patient education.

References

Aaronson, N.K., Bartelink, H., van Dongen, J.A. & van Dam, J. (1988) Evaluation of breast concerning therapy: clinical methodological and psychological perspectives. *European Journal of Surgical Oncology*, **14**, 133–40.

Agresti, A. (1984) *Analysis of Original Categorical Data.* Wiley & Sons, New York.

Agresti, A. (1990) *Categorical Data Analysis.* Wiley & Sons, New York.

Bartlett, E.E., Grayson, M., Barker, R., Levine, D.M., Golden, A. & Libber, S. (1984) The effects of physician communication skills on patient satisfaction; recall, and adherence. *Journal of Chronic Diseases*, **37**, 755–64.

Blanchard, C.G., Labrecque, M.S., Ruckdeschel, J.C. & Blanchard, E.B. (1988) Information and decision-making preferences of hospitalized adult cancer patients. *Social Science and Medicine*, **27**, 1139–45.

Bubela, N., Galloway, S., McCay, E., McKibbon, A., Nagle, L., Pringle, D. *et al.* (1990) Factors influencing patients' informational needs at time of hospital discharge. *Patient Education and Counselling*, **16**, 21–8.

Cassileth, B.R., Zupkis, R.V., Sutton-Smith, K. & March, V. (1980) Information and participation preferences among cancer patients. *Annals of Internal Medicine*, **92**, 832–6.

Cawley, M., Kostic, J. & Cappelo, C. (1990) Informational and psychosocial needs of women choosing conservative surgery/primary radiation for early stage breast cancer. *Cancer Nursing*, **13**, 90–94.

Close, A. (1988) Patient education: a literature view. *Journal of Advanced Nursing*, **13**, 203–13.

Comstock, L.M., Hooper, E.M., Goodwin, J.M. & Goodwin, J.S. (1982) Physician behaviours that correlate with patient satisfaction. *Journal of Medical Education*, **57**, 105–12.

Derdiarian, A. (1986) Informational needs of recently diagnosed cancer patients. *Nursing Research*, **35**, 276–81.

Dodd, M.J. (1988) The efficacy of pro-active information on self care in chemotherapy patients. *Patient Education and Counseling*, **11**, 215–25.

Fredette, S.L. (1990) A model for improving cancer patient education. *Cancer Nursing*, **13**, 207–15.

Fredette, S.L. & Beattie, H.M. (1986) Living with cancer. A patient education program. *Cancer Nursing*, **9**, 308–16.

Givio, J. (1986) What doctors tell patients with breast cancer about diagnosis and treatment: Findings from a study in general hospitals. *British Journal of Cancer*, **54**, 319–26.

Graydon, J.E. (1994) Women with breast cancer: their quality of life following a course of radiation therapy. *Journal of Advanced Nursing*, **19**, 617–22.

Hack, T.F., Degner, L.F. & Dyck, D.G. (1994) Relationship between preferences for decisional control and illness information among women with breast cancer: a quantitative and qualitative analysis. *Social Science and Medicine*, **39**, 279–89.

Hailey, B.J., Lavine, B. & Hogan, B. (1988) The mastectomy experience: patients' perspectives. *Women and Health*, **14**, 75–88.

Hakulinen, T., Kenward, M. & Luostarinen, T. (1989) *Cancer in Finland in 1954–2008: Incidence, Mortality and Prevalence by Region*. Cancer Society, Helsinki, Finland.

Harrison-Woermke, D.E. & Graydon, J.E. (1993) Perceived informational needs of breast cancer patients receiving radiation therapy after excisional biopsy and axillary node dissection. *Cancer Nursing*, an international journal for Cancer Care, **16**, 449–55.

Hartfield, M.J., Cason, C.L. & Cason, G.J. (1982) The effect of information about a threatening procedure on patient's expectations and emotional distress. *Nursing Research*, **31**, 202–5.

Krantz, D.S., Baum, A. & Wideman, M. (1980) Assessment of preferences for self-treatment and information in health care. *Journal of Personality and Social Psychology*, **39**, 977–90.

Larson, P.J. (1984) Important nurse caring behaviours perceived by patients with cancer. *Oncology Nursing Forum*, **11**, 46–50.

Lazarus, R. Folkman, S. (1984) *Stress, Appraisal and Coping*. Springer, New York.

Leino-Kilpi, H. (1990) Good nursing care. On what basis? Annales Universitatis Turkuensis. Ser. D. *Medica-Odontologica*, **49**. Turku University, Turku, Finland.

Lerman, C., Daly, M., Walsh, W.P., Resch, N., Seay, J., Barsevick, A., Birenbaum, L., Heggan, T. & Martin, G. (1993) Communication between patients with breast cancer and health care providers. Determinants and implications. *Cancer*, **72**, 2612–20.

Lindsey, A.M., Norbeck, J.S., Carrieri, V.L. & Perry, E. (1981) Social support and health outcomes in postmastectomy women: a review. *Cancer Nursing*, **4**, 377–84.

Mackillop, W.J., Stewart, W.E., Ginsburg, A.D. & Stewart, S.S. (1988) Cancer patients' perceptions of their disease and its treatment. *British Journal of Cancer*, **58**, 355–8.

Mishel, M.H. (1984) Perceived uncertainty as a stress in illness. *Research in Nursing and Health*, **7**, 163–71.

Molleman, E., Krabbendam, P.J., Annyas, A.A., Koops, H.S., Sleijfer, D.T. & Vermey, A. (1984) The significance of the doctor–patient relationship in coping with cancer. *Social Science and Medicine*, **18**, 475–80.

Neufeld, K.R., Degner, L.F. & Dick, J.A. (1993) A nursing intervention strategy to foster patient involvement in treatment decisions. *Oncology Nursing Forum*, **20**, 631–5.

Northouse, L.L. & Swain, M.A. (1987) Adjustment of patients and husbands to the initial impact of breast cancer. *Nursing Research*, **36**, 221–5.

Oberst, M.T. & James, R. (1985) Going home: patient and spouse adjustment following cancer surgery. *Topics in Clinical Nursing*, **7**, 46–75.

Padilla, G.V., Grant, M.M., Rains, B.L., Henson, B., Bergstrom, N., Wong, D. *et al.* (1981) Distress reduction and the effects of preparatory teaching films and patient control. *Research in Nursing and Health*, **4**, 375–87.

Pender, N.J. (1974) Patient identification of health information received during hospitalization. *Nursing Research*, **23**, 262–7.

Pfefferbaum, B. & Levenson, P.M. (1982) Adolescent cancer patient and physician responses to a questionnaire on patient concerns. *American Journal of Psychiatry*, **139**, 348–51.

Plant, H., Richardson, J., Stubbs, L., Lynch, D., Ellwood, J., Slevin, M. *et al.* (1987) Evaluation of a support group for cancer patients and their families and friends. *British Journal of Hospital Medicine*, **30**, 317–22.

Pukkala, E., Rimpelä, A. & Läärä, E. (1987) *Cancer in Finland.* Register for Cancer Patients in Finland, Helsinki, Finland.

Pålsson, M-B. & Norberg, A. (1995) Breast cancer patients' experiences of nursing care with the focus on emotional support: the implementation of a nursing intervention. *Journal of Advanced Nursing*, **21**, 277–85.

Schain, W.S., d'Angelo, T.M., Dunn, M.E., Lichter, A.S. & Pierce, L.J. (1994) Mastectomy versus conservative surgery and radiation therapy. Psychosocial consequences. *Cancer*, **73**, 1221–8.

Sime, A.M. & Libera, M.B. (1985) Relationship of preoperative fear, type of coping and information received about surgery to recovery from surgery. *Journal of Personality and Social Psychology*, **34**, 716–24.

Summers, R. (1984) Should patients be told more? *Nursing Mirror*, **159**, 16–20.

Tilley, J.D., Gregor, F.M. & Thiesson, V. (1987) The nurse's role in patient education: incongruent perceptions among nurses and patients. *Journal of Advanced Nursing*, **12**, 291–301.

Ward, S. & Griffin, J. (1990) Developing a test of knowledge of surgical options for breast cancer. *Cancer Nursing*, **13**, 191–6.

Willits, M.J. (1994) Role of 'Reach of Recovery' in breast cancer. *Cancer*, **74**, 2172–2173.

Wilson-Barnett, J. (1988) Patient teaching or patient counselling? *Journal of Advanced Nursing*, **13**, 215–22.

Wilson-Barnett, J. & Osborne, J. (1983) Studies evaluating patient teaching: implications for practice. *International Journal of Nursing Studies*, **20**, 33–44.

Ziemer, M.M. (1983) Effects of information on post surgical coping. *Nursing Research*, **32**, 282–7.

Chapter 7
Evaluation of the pain response by Mexican American and Anglo American women and their nurses

EVELYN RUIZ CALVILLO, *RN, DNSc*
Professor, Department of Nursing, California State University, Los Angeles, California, USA

and JACQUELYN H. FLASKERUD, *RN, PhD*
Professor, School of Nursing, University of California, Los Angeles, California, USA

This study examined the relationship between ethnicity and pain. The study addressed three major research questions. The first question asked whether there was a significant difference in Mexican American women's and Anglo American women's response to cholecystectomy pain. Secondly, the nurses' attribution of pain to each of the two ethnic groups was compared. Finally, the patient's evaluation of the pain being experienced was compared to the nurse's evaluation of the pain the patient was experiencing. The sample consisted of 60 patient subjects and 60 nurse responses. Data were collected at two major teaching hospitals in southern California, USA. Patient pain was measured using the McGill Pain Questionnaire, amount of analgesics and three physiological measures. The nurse's assessment of patient pain was measured using the Present Pain Intensity scale. MANOVA was used to analyse differences between the two ethnic groups on all measures of pain and no significant differences were found between the two ethnic groups on any of the measures of pain. However, nurses judged the two ethnic groups' pain response differently, assigning more pain to Anglo Americans. Finally, a dependent t-test was used to compare nurses' and patients' evaluation of pain. There were significant differences. Nurses evaluated the patient's pain as being less than patients did. Pearson product-moment correlations were used to examine the relationship between pain and sample characteristics of both patients and nurses. For the nurses, pain was significantly related to the patient's education, place of birth, language and religion.

Introduction

In each culture there is a way of life within which an individual may acquire attitudes, values, religious practices, language, and so on, as well as responses to pain, fear, and other emotional responses. Whether a person is more or less sensitive to pain or expresses a certain response to pain may depend, among other factors, on whether that individual's culture values or devalues the display of emotional expression and response to illness and injury.

Management of pain and societal response to an individual's expression of pain may also be culturally determined. When the person experiencing pain and the caregiver share the same values regarding the expression of pain, there may be little conflict over its management. However, when caregiver and patient differ in their attitudes toward the perception and expression of pain, problems may occur for both patient and caregiver. Sometimes this difference may be attributed to cultural differences. At other times, it may be attributed to the differences in professional and lay-person attitudes toward pain.

This study focused on two major variables, ethnicity and pain, and on how Mexican American and Anglo American women respond to postoperative cholecystectomy pain. In addition, the study focused on the evaluation of the pain response by the patient and the nursing staff. The purpose of the study was to describe and compare the effect that ethnicity has on the postoperative experience of Mexican American and Anglo American women and to provide information useful for the assessment of the pain experience. A second purpose was to describe and compare lay (patient) and professional (nurse) perceptions of pain.

Literature review

Factors influencing the pain response

According to Melzack (1975, 1983), pain is not just a physiological response to tissue damage but also includes behavioural and emotional responses expected and accepted by one's cultural group which may influence the perception of pain. These expectations are stored in the brain and in cultural experiences and are capable of influencing the transmission of painful stimuli throughout the individual's life. When pain is occurring, physiological processes as well as the individual's thoughts, cultural beliefs and values, and memories can influence whether pain impulses reach the level of awareness (Meinhart & McCaffery 1983).

Perception, expression and management of pain are all embedded in a cultural context. The definition of pain, just like that of health and illness, is culturally determined (Ludwig-Beymer 1989). According to Meinhart & McCaffery (1983) cultural expectations may specify:

(1) Different reactions according to age, sex and occupation.
(2) What treatment to seek.
(3) The intensity and duration of pain that should be tolerated.
(4) What responses should be made.
(5) Who to report to when pain occurs.
(6) What types of pain require attention.

It is possible that a patient's cultural background influences not only attitudes towards pain but the overt response to it as well.

Several other psychological and social conditions have been related to the pain response. These conditions include anxiety, self-esteem, social support and sick-role adaptation (Berkman 1984; Davitz & Davitz 1981; Dunn 1976; Fordyce *et al.* 1984; Turk *et al.* 1983). Relationships between pain and each of these concepts have been proposed. Anxiety is thought to increase the pain experienced; a direct relationship is proposed between pain intensity and anxiety. Social support, self-esteem and sick-role adaptation are thought to buffer the pain experience; inverse relationships between pain intensity and self-esteem, social support and sick-role adaptation are proposed.

Pain response in Anglo Americans

Anglo American refers to white non-Hispanic people of European origin of more than two generations living in the United States. Anglo Americans are frequently selected as the reference group in cross-cultural comparison studies because their social and cultural behaviours represent the accepted pattern (Castro *et al.* 1984; Winsberg & Greenlick 1967; Zborowski 1952, 1969). Their beliefs are considered dominant in spite of the fact that there is little social research done on Anglo Americans (Harwood 1981).

Zborowski (1952, 1969) conducted the best-known study of pain in various ethnic groups. The study described the dominant culture values of pain experience which are still used today. The Anglo American patient reports pain and is able to give a detailed description of it; however, the person usually demonstrates few emotional reactions to pain. When in pain, the Anglo American tries to remain calm avoiding complaining, crying, screaming, or other manifestations of pain. According to Meinhart & McCaffery (1983), stoicism is valued by Anglo Americans; there is pride in being the good patient, i.e. one who does not annoy anyone with his or her pain experience.

Zborowski's early study has been pertinent to subsequent cross-cultural studies on the influence of culture on pain. He suggested that patterned attitudes toward pain exist in every culture. Appropriate and inappropriate expressions of pain are culturally prescribed. Cultural traditions dictate whether to expect and tolerate pain in certain situations and how to behave during a painful experience (Ludwig-Beymer 1989).

Hospital staff in Zborowski's study tended to support the 'Old American' (Anglo-Saxon) response to pain and to characterize the other groups as over-reacting, emotional and complaining. Zborowski disagreed with this interpretation considering it too simplistic. He reached two conclusions based on his study:

(1) Similar reactions (behaviours, vocalizations) to pain demonstrated by members of different ethnocultural groups do not necessarily reflect similar attitudes toward pain.
(2) Reactive patterns similar in their manifestations (e.g. crying, moaning or stoicism) may have different functions in various cultures (Zborowski 1952).

Pain response in Mexican Americans

Calatrello (1980) examined the traditional health beliefs of Hispanics. In many Hispanic cultures the value of suffering and the concept of fatalism are accepted beliefs with religious undertones. One's fate is to suffer in this world and 'submit with patience to one's allotted measure of suffering' (Calatrello 1980). When an individual is ill, the person bears the illness with dignity and courage; this is because many Hispanics believe that difficulties are part of life and must be accepted without complaint. Stoicism is valued, and often signs and symptoms of pain are not acknowledged because lack of stamina is considered a sign of weakness.

Many Mexican American patients, especially women, moan when uncomfortable. Consequently, they are often identified by the nursing staff as complainers who cannot tolerate pain (Orque *et al.* 1983). These investigators have stated that, in the Mexican culture, crying out in response to pain is an acceptable expression and not synonymous with an inability to tolerate pain. Crying out does not necessarily indicate either that the pain experience is severe or that the person is experiencing a loss of self-control. Neither does it mean that the patient expects the nurse to intervene. In the Mexican culture, the pattern of crying and moaning may have the function for the patient of relieving pain rather than the function of communicating a request for intervention.

In cross-cultural studies which included Hispanic subjects, differences were found between them, Anglo Americans, and other ethnic/racial groups in how patients viewed and described their pain (Kalish & Reynolds 1976; Meinhart & McCaffery 1983). The descriptions by the Hispanic subjects were consistent with the beliefs of fatalism, stoicism and self-restraint reported as valued in the Hispanic culture.

In a study conducted by Lipton & Marbach (1980), ethnic differences in 166 patients with chronic facial pain of unknown origin were studied. The groups included Hispanic, black, Jewish and white Catholic and Protestant patients. The emotional response to pain such as tears and moans was similar but there were distinct differences in how patients viewed and described their pain. In the study, Hispanics were less willing to admit loss of control and less likely to describe their pain as unbearable. Despite these consistent findings, the belief persists among Anglo health care workers that Hispanics are dramatic complainers who have a low tolerance for pain (Perez-Stable 1987).

Evaluation of pain response by nurses

Health caregivers' views of pain have been analysed in many studies in which the culture of the patient and the nurse did not differ or in which culture was not considered as a variable. There have been consistent differences between patients and staff in assessing the severity of patients' pain (Melzack *et al.* 1987; Teske *et al.* 1983). Among studies of nurses, it has been shown that the nurses' perceptions of pain did not coincide with the patients, which generally resulted in more suffering for the patient (Cohen 1980; Jacox 1979; Teske *et al.* 1983). Regardless of culture, nurses gave less medication for pain than ordered and less medication than patients needed to alleviate their pain. The goal of the nurses was to reduce the patients' pain, not to relieve it (Rankin & Snider 1984).

Dudley & Holm (1984) found that nurses tended to infer a greater degree of psychological distress than pain. They made the observation that such an inference can lead to inappropriate management of suffering; that is, patients will be given psychological support but not pain intervention.

Staff views of pain have been reported in many cross-cultural studies. These studies confirm that medical and nursing personnel underestimate patients' pain and limit analgesics (Streltzer & Wade 1981; Winsberg & Greenlick 1967). Nursing staff tended to uphold the dominant cultural values which strongly encourage stoicism during pain experiences and to believe that patients exaggerate their pain experiences.

Davitz & Davitz (1981) studied nurses' attitudes toward pain and found that the patient's ethnicity was related to how much physical and psychological distress the nurse believed the patient was experiencing. Nurses thought that Jewish and Spanish-speaking patients expressed the most distress with pain and Anglo-Saxon patients the least. The nurses' own cultural background also influenced how much distress they thought patients were experiencing with pain. Nurses of Northern European and United States background thought patients were experiencing less physical pain and psychological distress, whereas nurses of Eastern and Southern European or African backgrounds thought patients were experiencing more pain and psychological distress. This was true regardless of the nurses' years of experience, position and area of practice. These investigators concluded that nurses' judgements about the pain and distress suffered by patients are influenced by their own beliefs about suffering.

Research questions

Three major research questions were addressed.

(1) Are there differences in the pain response of Mexican American and Anglo American women who have had an elective cholecystectomy?
(2) Are there differences in the pain response of Mexican American and Anglo American women as evaluated by the nurse?
(3) Are there differences between the patient and the nurse in the evaluation of the patient's pain response?

Two additional questions were asked.

(1) Are there differences between the two groups in acculturation, anxiety, self-esteem, social support and functional independence?
(2) What is the relationship of the pain response to social support, self-esteem, anxiety, functional independence and sociodemographic characteristics?

Instruments

The variables of interest in the study were pain, culture, anxiety, self-esteem, social support and functional independence. The intruments chosen to measure these variables had all previously demonstrated reliability and validity. Each variable was measured using at least two instruments to establish construct validity. Content validity of instruments was established by an expert panel of judges. Reliability of each instrument was established using test–retest, alternative form, or Cronbach's alpha coefficient as a measure of internal consistency. Using these psychometric measures, all instruments were judged to have acceptable levels of reliability and validity for this study (Calvillo & Flaskerud 1993). All instruments were administered by the principal investigator.

Elective cholecystectomy

Elective cholecystectomy was chosen as the pain stimulus. It was assumed that cholecystectomy surgery would present a similar stimulus to all patients.

Pain was measured on the second postoperative day using the McGill pain questionnaire (MPQ) (Melzack 1975, 1983), the amount of analgesics received on the day of surgery and the first two postoperative days was measured (American Pain Society 1989; Scott *et al.* 1983; McCaffery & Beebe 1989), and pulse, respiration and blood pressure measured preoperatively and the second postoperative day (McGuire 1984; Waltz *et al.* 1984). The nurse's evaluation of pain was measured using the present pain intensity scale of the MPQ on the second postoperative day (Melzack 1975, 1983).

The MPQ collects data on the pain rating index (PRI-T), the number of words chosen (NWC), and the present pain intensity scale (PPI). Cronbach's alpha coefficient for PRI-T was 0.83. Alternative form reliability for the PRI-T and the PPI was $r = 0.73$, $P = 0.0001$; for PRI-T and NWC, $r = 0.89$, $P = 0.0001$; and for NWC and PPI was $r = 0.64$, $P = 0.0001$. The amount of pain medication given to each patient was calculated to equal doses of morphine 10 mg by use of the equinalgesic chart (McCaffery & Beebe 1989). The PPI correlation with amount of medication for day three was $r = 0.65$, $P = 0.0001$. None of the parts of the MPQ correlated with blood pressure, pulse and respirations taken on the day pain was evaluated (the second postoperative day).

Culture

Culture was measured preoperatively by the acculturation scale and by self-identification as a member of either the Mexican American or Anglo American ethnic group. The acculturation scale measures level of acculturation based on several measures of language preference and social relationships (Marin *et al.* 1987). The Cronbach's alpha coefficient for the acculturation scale was 0.90.

Anxiety was measured preoperatively and the second postoperative day by the state-trait anxiety inventory (Cronbach's alpha = 0.93 and 0.91, respectively) (Spielberger & Diaz-Guererro 1976). Self-esteem was measured the second postoperative day by the self-esteem inventory (alpha = 0.89) (Coopersmith 1967). Social support was measured on the second postoperative day by the social support scale (alpha = 0.77) (Nyamathi & Flaskerud 1992, Zich & Temoshok 1987). Finally, functional independence was measured on the second postoperative day by the activities of daily living scale (alpha = 0.83) (Bernier & Small 1988, Katz *et al.* 1963).

Sociodemographic characteristics of patient subjects measured were age, income, education, marital status, number of children, occupation, religion, place of birth, number of previous hospitalizations and number of previous surgeries. Nurse sample characteristics measured were age, ethnicity, place of birth, basic nursing education, and years of experience in nursing.

Methodology

The study design was descriptive, correlational and comparative. it was conducted on surgical units in two large university teaching hospitals in southern California which serve large percentages of Mexican American and Anglo American patients.

Sample

Patients

Sixty patients participated in the study. They were selected for an interview and chosen on the basis of the following criteria:

(1) Women identified as either Mexican American or Anglo American (white non-Hispanic).
(2) Scheduled for an elective cholecystectomy by an abdominal incision. Patients who had the gallbladder removed by laporoscopic incisions were excluded. Any patient whose recovery was complicated was excluded as the study progressed. Complications included infection, haemorrhage, obstruction of the T-tube if one was present, respiratory complications, circulatory complications, or cancer. Patients having an emergency cholecystectomy were not considered. Patients having incidental appendectomies were included but all other surgery combinations were excluded.

When sample criteria were met, the patient was asked by the investigator whether she was interested in being involved in the study. A verbal explanation of the study was given by the investigator. The patient was given at least 10 minutes for consideration. If the patient was willing to participate, the consent forms were read and signed and the preoperative instruments were administered. Sample characteristics are displayed in Table 7.1.

Chi-square analysis ($P < 0.05$) was used to determine the relationship between ethnicity and each of the sociodemographic characteristics. There were no significant relationships between ethnicity and age, number of children, and occupation. There were significant relationships between ethnicity and place of birth, marital status, education, religion, number of hospitalizations, number of surgeries, and family income. Anglo Americans had more education and higher income. However, the entire sample might be characterized as low to middle income. Mexican Americans were more often married, Catholic, born outside the US, and had more previous hospitalizations and surgeries.

Table 7.1 Sample characteristics for the two ethnic groups.

Characteristics	Mexican American (n = 22)		Anglo American (n = 38)	
Place of birth	Mexico	(73%)	US	(100%)
Age ($\bar{x}$)	35 years		37 years	
Marital status	Married	(45%)	Married	(50%)
Children ($\bar{x}$)	2		2	
Education	⩽ 8th grade	(41%)	High school	(50%)
Occupation	Housewife	(64%)	Housewife	(42%)
Family income	< $20 000	(77%)	< $20 000	(62%)
Religion	Catholic	(77%)	Protestant	(66%)
Previous hospitalizations	82%		68%	
Previous surgeries	41%		28%	

Nurses

Nurses responsible for medicating the patients who agreed to participate in the study made up the nurse sample. While there were 32 nurses in the study, 60 nurse responses were recorded, one for each patient. Only those nurses on duty from 7.00 A.M. to 3.00 P.M. were asked to participate. Because each nurse may have been assigned to more than one patient in the study, a record was kept of the assignments. The assignments were monitored to ensure that the nurse did not exclusively nor consecutively complete the instruments for the same ethnic group. Two nurses in the study participated in four pain evaluations, five participated in three evaluations, 12 performed two evaluations, and the remaining 13 nurses participated in one each.

For the nurse subjects, years of experience in nursing ranged from 1 to 20 years, with a mean of 12 years; 31.7% had more than 12 years experience and 30% between 4 and 6 years. Basic nursing education was identified as 30.9% baccalaureate, 27.3% associate degree, 25.5% diploma, and 16.4% licensed vocational nurse. Age ranged from 22 to 58 years, with a mean of 42 years. The majority (71.7%) were born in the US. The rest (18.3%) were identified as from Hungary, England, Peru, the Philippines, Canada, San Salvador, China and Mexico. Ethnic groups identified were 45.8% Anglo American, 18.6% Asian American, 10.2% black American, 6.8% Mexican American, and the remainder other ethnicities.

Results

The first major research question asked whether there was a difference in pain response between Mexican American and Anglo American women.

Multiple analysis of variance (MANOVA) using the Hotelling–Lawley trace measure was used to examine differences in the two patient groups on each measure of pain. There were no significant differences in Mexican American and Anglo American women's response to cholecystectomy pain on any of the measures of pain (Table 7.2).

Table 7.2   Differences in pain between the two ethnic groups.

Measures of pain assessment	Mexican Americans ($n=22$) ($\bar{x}$)	Anglo Americans ($n=38$) ($\bar{x}$)	MANOVA		
			F	d.f.	P
McGill pain questionnaire					
Pain rating index – total	15.7	18.7	1.29	1,57	0.26
Number of words chosen	8.8	9.3	0.29	1,57	0.58
Present pain intensity	2.1	2.7	0.01	1,57	0.91
Pain medication					
Amount day 1	22.8	23.0	0.01	1,53	0.92
Amount day 2	32.9	31.0	0.16	1,53	0.69
Amount day 3	16.1	19.7	0.76	1,53	0.39
Vital signs					
Systolic blood pressure	121.3	126.9	2.38	1,58	0.13
Diastolic blood pressure	72.0	73.2	0.31	1,58	0.58
Pulse	82.3	81.2	0.11	1,58	0.74
Respirations	19.3	19.5	0.16	1,58	0.69

The second major research question addressed differences in the pain response for Mexican American and Anglo American women as assessed by the nurse. The mean score on the present pain intensity scale (PPI) as evaluated by the nurse for Mexican Americans was 1.1 and for Anglo Americans, was 1.6. There was a significant difference in pain scores between the two ethnic groups as evaluated by the nurse, with Anglo American patients assessed as experiencing more pain ($F = 4.16$; d.f. $= 1,57$; $P < 0.05$).

The final major research question focused on differences between patient and nurse assessment of patients' pain. A dependent t-test found significant differences between nurses' evaluation of pain using the PPI and the patients' evaluation of pain ($t = 6.63$; d.f. $= 1.57$; $P = 0.0001$). The mean for nurses was 0.75 and the mean for patients was 1.33 with patients assessing pain as more severe than nurses.

A secondary research question asked whether the two patient groups differed in acculturation, anxiety, self-esteem, social support and functional independence. Although the two patient groups were selected to represent two different ethnic and cultural groups, it was considered necessary to measure the presumed ethnic and cultural differences between the two patient groups. An analysis of variance was used to determine the relationship of ethnic group self-identity to acculturation scale score. There was a significant relationship between ethnic group identity and acculturation scale score (F = 62.51; d.f. = 1.44; $P < 0.0001$) establishing that the two groups actually did differ in ethnicity and level of acculturation.

Using repeated-measures analysis of variance, there were no significant differences between the two ethnic groups in state or trait anxiety over time. Univariate analysis of variance was used to examine differences between the two ethnic groups on self-esteem inventory scores, social support scores, and activities of daily living scores. There were no significant differences between the two patient/ethnic groups on any of these measures.

Other variables

Another secondary research question asked whether the pain response was related to the other variables of interest. Pearson product-moment correlation coefficients (r) were used to examine relationships between pain and anxiety, self-esteem, social support, and functional independence. Conceptually it was proposed that anxiety would increase pain and the other variables would decrease pain. There were significant inverse correlations between pain and anxiety ($r = -0.47$, $P = 0.0002$) and between pain and self-esteem ($r = -0.43$, $P = 0.0007$). Relationships between social support and pain and functional independence and pain were not significant. Only the relationship between pain and self-esteem was in the expected direction.

Sociodemographic characteristics

Finally, relationships were examined between patient sociodemographic characteristics and evaluation of pain using the PPI scores. There were no significant relationships between patients' evaluations of their pain and place of birth, age, marital status, number of children, education, occupation, family income, religion, number of previous hospitalizations, number of previous surgeries, and admission weight. In addition, the relationship between nurse sample characteristics and PPI scores were examined. There were no significant relationships between the nurses' PPI scores and their years of experience, type of nursing programme, ethnicity, and place of birth.

However, there were significant relationships between five patient characteristics and the nurse's evaluation of the patient's pain. Nurses judged patient's pain to be more severe for blue collar and professional occupations, for high school graduates and those with some college, for those born in the US, for those who spoke English, and for those whose religion was Protestant (Table 7.3).

Table 7.3 Significant relationships between patient characteristics and nurses' evaluation of their patients' pain.

Patient characteristic	Nurse PPI score		ANOVA		
	n	$\bar{x}$	F	d.f.	*P*
Occupation			4.05	3,51	0.01
Not working housewife	27	1.15			
Unskilled	10	1.00			
Blue collar	5	2.00			
Professional	13	1.95			
Education			3.56	3,56	0.02
8th grade or less	11	0.73			
Some high school	10	1.30			
High school graduate	25	1.56			
Some college/trade	14	1.80			
Birth place			2.95	16,42	0.02
US	43	1.60			
Mexico	17	0.94			
Language			3.18	17,41	0.01
English	42	1.61			
Spanish	18	0.94			
Religion			3.02	24,28	0.005
Catholic	29	1.17			
Protestant	25	1.68			

Discussion

Several investigators conducting cross-cultural studies have found differences in the pain response between groups related to ethnic or cultural variations. These studies concluded that culture and ethnicity played a role in pain behaviour (Lipton & Marbach 1980; Sternback & Tursky 1965; Zborowski 1952, 1969). However, other studies found no differences based on ethnicity (Flannery *et al.* 1981; Winsberg & Greenlick 1967). Importantly, both Hispanic Americans and Anglo Americans have been described in the literature as stoic in their response to pain (Calatrello 1980; Kalish & Reynolds 1976; Meinhart & McCaffery 1983; Zborowski 1952, 1969).

The findings of this study support these latter conclusions: no differences in the pain response were found between Mexican and Anglo American subjects. Both groups responded to pain in what might be considered a stoic or understated manner: they judged pain as 'discomforting', a '2' on a scale from 0 to 5.

It is possible that patients under-rated their pain. Many factors influence patients to undercomplain. Patients may not discuss their pain with nurses or physicians because of fears such as addiction or a perception that health care workers will respond negatively to requests for pain medication. In addition, patients may be reluctant to admit to pain because this may signal a worsening of their condition, a fear perhaps developed as members of a particular culture.

Patient ethnicity

The findings of this study, that nurses judge patients' pain differently based on patient ethnicity, is supported by the literature (Winsberg & Greenlick 1967; Zborowski 1952, 1969). In this study, nurses evaluated Anglo American women's pain as more severe than Mexican American women's pain. However, the literature focuses more on the nurse's characterization or stereotype of the expression or reaction to pain by each ethnic group.

A major finding of this study is that nurses are assigning more pain to Anglo and to 'higher' social-class patients: those who were more educated, had professional or skilled occupations, spoke English, and were born in the US. It might be assumed that patients with these social-class characteristics would also receive more pain management, more attention, and more pain relief than other patients. This finding might be interpreted cautiously, that nurses assign a greater amount of pain and more credibility to the expression of pain to those patients with more social value.

Another explanation for the difference may be attributed to the ability of these patients to communicate to the nurse that pain was occurring. Mexican patients with less education and poor English skills may have had difficulty communicating pain severity, resulting in lower scores given by their nurses.

Different assessments of pain

Finally, the finding that nurses and patients assess patients' pain differently is supported overwhelmingly in the literature (Dudley & Holm 1984; Miller & Jay 1985; Teske *et al.* 1983). In all studies cited, patients evaluated their pain as more severe than nurses. This study supported that same conclusion. Nurses evaluated pain as less for all patients, scoring patient pain as 'mild' or a '1' on the PPI scale (0 to 5 range) while patients scored their pain as 'discomforting' or a '2' on the PPI scale.

The study was limited by small sample size, purposive sampling, the setting in two hospitals in southern California, and pain related to a single source. Possible threats to validity include the hospital environment and the testing situation.

Implications for nursing

The findings highlight the need for nurses to be more aware that their own values and perceptions may affect how they evaluate the patient's response to pain and ultimately how that pain is treated. To avoid potential mis-interpretation that could lead to inadequate evaluation and control of pain, validation with the patient is necessary. When a patient requests pain medication, validation can be ensured by concurrent evaluation of the pain by both the patient and the nurse.

Future studies are needed not only between the two patient groups in this study but with other cultural groups. Studies that focus on the meaning of pain for individuals in different cultures would increase understanding of pain perception. Some research has been conducted with a focus on the effect the nurse's culture has on pain evaluation; the findings in this study point to the need for additional research in this area. How nurses perceive and evaluate pain during various other clinical conditions is another area of research important to nursing practice.

Acknowledgements

This study was supported in part by the Dissertation Year Fellowship, UCLA, and the Minority Faculty Award, CSULA. Professor Calvillo was a doctoral candidate at UCLA when these data were collected.

References

American Pain Society (1989) *Principles of Analgesic Use in Treatment of Acute Pain and Chronic Cancer Pain: A Concise Guide to Medical Practice.* American Pain Society, Washington, DC.

Berkman, L.F. (1984) Assessing the physical health effects of social networks and social support. *Annual Review of Public Health,* **5**, 413–32.

Bernier, S.L. & Small, N.R. (1988) Disruptive behaviours. *Journal of Gerontological Nursing,* **14**(2), 8–13.

Calatrello, R.L. (1980) The hispanic concept of illness: an obstacle to effective healthcare management? *Behavioral Medicine,* **7**(11), 23–28.

Calvillo, E.R. & Flaskerud, J.H. (1993) The adequacy and scope of the Roy Adaptation Model to guide cross-cultural pain research. *Nursing Science Quarterly,* **6**(3), 118–29.

Castro, F.G., Furth, P. & Karlow, H. (1984) The health beliefs of Mexican, Mexican American, and Anglo American women. *Hispanic Journal of Behavioral Sciences,* **6**(4), 365–86.

Cohen, F.L. (1980) Postsurgical pain relief. Patients' status and nurses' medication choices. *Pain,* **9**(1), 265–74.

Coopersmith, S. (1967) *The Antecedents of Self-Esteem.* W.H. Freeman and Company, San Francisco.

Davitz, J.R. & Davitz, L.J. (1981) *Influences on Patients' Pain and Psychological Distress.* Springer-Verlag, New York.

Dudley, S.R. & Holm, K. (1984) Assessment of the pain experience in relation to selected nurse characteristics. *Pain,* **18**(2), 179–86.

Dunn, J.R. (1976) Regulation of the senses. In *Introduction to Nursing: An Adaptation Model* (Ed. C. Roy), pp. 133–150. Prentice-Hall, Englewood Cliffs, New Jersey.

Flannery, R.B., Sos, J. & McGovern, P. (1981) Ethnicity as a factor in the expression of pain. *Psychosomatics,* **22**(1), 34–9, 45, 49–50.

Fordyce, W.E., Lansky, D., Calsyn, D.A., Shelton, J.L., Stolov, W.C. & Rock, D.L. (1984) Pain measurement and pain behavior. *Pain*, **18**, 53–69.

Harwood, A. (1981) *Ethnicity and Medical Care.* Harvard University Press, Cambridge, Massachusetts.

Jacox, A.K. (1979) Assessing pain. *American Journal of Nursing*, **79**(5), 894–900.

Kalish, R.A. & Reynolds, D.K. (1976) *Death and Ethnicity: A Psycho-Cultural Study.* Ethel Percy Andrus Gerontology Center/University of Southern California, Los Angeles.

Katz, S., Ford, A.B., Moskowitz, R.W., Jackson, B.A. & Jaffe, M.W. (1963) The index of ADL: a standardized measure of biological and psychosocial function. *Journal of the American Medical Association*, **185**(12), 94–9.

Lipton, J.S. & Marbach, J.J. (1980) Pain differences, similarities found. *Science News*, **118**, 182–3.

Ludwig-Beymer, P. (1989) Transcultural aspects of pain. In *Transcultural Concepts in Nursing Care* (Eds J.S. Boyle & M.M. Andrews). Scott-Foresman, Glenview, Illinois.

Marin, G., Sabogal, F., Marin, B., Otero-Sabogal, R. & Perez-Stable, E.J. (1987) Development of a short acculturation scale for hispanics. *Hispanic Journal of Behavior Sciences*, **9**(2), 183–205.

McCaffery, M. & Beebe, A. (1989) *Pain Clinical Manual for Nursing Practice.* C.V. Mosby, St Louis.

McGuire, D.B. (1984) The measurement of clinical pain. *Nursing Research*, **33**(3), 152–6.

Meinhart, N.T. & McCaffery, M. (1983) *Pain: A Nursing Approach to Assessment and Analysis.* Appleton-Century-Crofts, Norwalk, Connecticut.

Melzack, R. (1975) McGill pain questionnaire: major properties and scoring methods. *Pain*, **1**, 277–99.

Melzack, R. (1983) *Pain Measurement and Assessment.* Raven Press, New York.

Melzack, R., Abbott, F.V., Zackon, W., Milder, D.S. & Davis, M.W.L. (1987) Pain on a surgical ward: a survey of the duration and intensity of pain and the effectiveness of medication. *Pain*, **29**, 67–72.

Miller, T.W. & Jay, L.L. (1985) Cognitive-behavioral and pharmaceutical approaches to sensory pain management. *Topics in Clinical Nursing*, **6**(4), 34–43.

Nyamathi, A. & Flaskerud, J.H. (1992) A community-based inventory of current concerns of impoverished homeless and drug addicted minority women. *Research in Nursing and Health*, **15**(2), 121–29.

Orque, M., Bloch, B. & Monrroy, L.S. (1983) *Ethnic Nursing Care: A Multicultural Approach.* C.V. Mosby, St. Louis.

Perez-Stable, E.J. (1987) Issues in Latino healthcare. *Western Journal of Medicine*, **139**, 820–28.

Rankin, M.A. & Snider, B. (1984) Nurse's perception of cancer patients' pain. *Cancer Nursing*, **7**(2), 149–55.

Scott, L.E., Chum, G.A. & Peoples, J.B. (1983) Preoperative predictors of postoperative pain. *Pain*, **15**(3), 283–93.

Spielberger, C.D. & Diaz-Guerrero, R. (eds) (1976) *Cross-Cultural Anxiety.* Hemisphere, Washington, DC.

Sternbach, R.A. & Tursky, B. (1965) Ethnic differences among housewives in psychophysical and skin potential responses to electric shock. *Psychophysiology*, **1**, 241–6.

Streltzer, J. & Wade, T.C. (1981) The influence of cultural group on the undertreatment of postoperative pain. *Psychosomatic Medicine*, **43**(5), 397–403.

Teske, K., Daut, R.L. & Cleeland, C.S. (1983) Relationships between nurses' observations and patients' self-reports of pain. *Pain*, **16**(3), 286–96.

Turk, D.C., Meichenbaum, D. & Genest, M. (1983) *Pain and Behavioral Medicine: A Cognitive-Behavioral Perspective.* Guilford Press, New York.

Waltz, C.F., Strickland, O.L. & Lenz, E.R. (1984) *Measurement in Nursing Research.* F.A. Davis, Philadelphia.

Winsberg, B. & Greenlick, M. (1967) Pain response in Negro and White obstetrical patients. *Journal of Health Social and Behavior*, **8**, 222–7.

Zborowski, M. (1952) Cultural components in responses to pain. *Journal of Social Issues*, **8**, 16–30.

Zborowski, M. (1969) *People in Pain*. Jossey-Bass, San Francisco.

Zich, J. & Temoshok, L. (1987) Perceptions of social support in men with AIDS and ARC: relationships with distress and hardiness. *Journal of Applied Social Psychology*, **17**(3), 193–215.

Chapter 8
Does the use of an assessment tool in the accident and emergency department improve the quality of care?

JANE CHRISTIE, *RN, RCNT, DipN, BSc(Hons), PGDE, MSc*
Lecturer Practitioner – Trauma Services, Oxford Radcliffe Hospital, Oxford, England

The aim of this study was to evaluate the effect of introducing a nursing record, using the SOAPE model, in the accident and emergency department. A working group was formed to design and implement a new record and evaluate its effect. A six-month teaching programme was run to prepare staff. Quality of documentation was measured using the Phaneuf audit tool both before and after the implementation of the new record and the teaching sessions. The results were compared. It was concluded that, overall, the documentation showed significant improvement. Therefore, it could be assumed that there had been an improvement in the quality of care.

Introduction

The importance of documentation has been a long-standing issue in nursing (Gropper 1988). Records provide written evidence of nursing practice, communication about patients' status, response to intervention and a measurement of the quality of care given (Tapp 1990). Legally, if what nurses do is not documented, it is not done (Sklar 1984; Hershey & Lawrence 1986; Cowan 1987; Morrissey-Ross 1988).

Despite the publication of a detailed report by the World Health Organization (WHO 1983) regarding the aims, methods, principles and recommendations for record writing, difficulties still persist. Nurses openly acknowledge problems with accuracy, completeness and timeliness (Gay 1983; Costello & Summers 1985; Morgan 1985; Tapp 1990). When nursing care activities are intense, nurses devalue documentation in favour of patient care (Harris 1979; Vasey 1979; Tapp 1990).

These problems are particularly prevalent in the accident and emergency (A/E) setting where the variety of symptoms or injuries, length of stay, peaks and troughs and a strong influence of the medical model leaves record-keeping as secondary importance (Bradley 1985). Documentation may often be left incomplete or, when records are written, they reflect a task-orientated approach to care with little attention paid to individual needs (Ruth 1986).

The purpose of this study was to introduce and evaluate a nursing assessment tool that would facilitate documentation of care in an accident and emergency department.

Literature review

On reviewing the literature it is evident that the writing of nursing records is an integral part of patient care and has been addressed by many (De La Cuesta 1983; WHO 1983; Walton 1986).

Reasons for documenting care

The WHO (1983) believed that by sharing information through records nurses would improve the standard and continuity of patient care, learn more about individual health needs and be able to participate in multi-disciplinary team conferences. During the 1970s, there was a realization that traditional approaches had limitations and that a systematic, evaluative approach was needed (Robinson 1990). Over the years documentation has changed to reflect the social climate (De la Cuesta 1983).

The WHO (1983) identifies the key reasons for documenting care as:

(1) A means of communicating care.
(2) A process of continuity, efficiency and measure of quality.
(3) A mechanism for accountability.
(4) A legal requirement.
(5) A method of expanding knowledge of the science of nursing.

Walton (1986) suggests that the aim of documentation is to facilitate improved communication and co-ordination of care to ensure each patient's needs are met and to demonstrate for legal and manpower planning purposes whether or not this has been achieved.

Records provide evidence of actions, reactions and goal achievement and they give direction for problem-solving (Yura & Walsh 1988; Sutcliffe 1990). They should provide a comprehensive picture of the patient's response to therapy, including observation and doctors' orders (Sklar 1984).

Calley & Siler (1987) believe that documenting problem-identification and problem-solving abilities are critical in demonstrating that nurses are responsible and accountable. Records put the onus on the caregiver to communicate; if there is no record then it could be assumed that no care was given (Morrissey-Ross 1988; Yura & Walsh 1988; Schmidt *et al.* 1990).

Records are legal documents and are the property of the Secretary of State (Cowan 1987). Nurses are legally bound to document their actions and, ultimately, nursing entries can substantially bolster the defence or render it useless (Sklar 1984). Documentation brings to the nursing profession dynamism and a spirit of creativity, it provides foundation for organizational change, personal development and professional growth and it can act as a tool to educate professionals in the expanding science of nursing (WHO 1983). The communication of professional practice, through documentation, can enhance professionalism (Fox-Ungar *et al.* 1989).

Process of documenting care

The WHO (1983) believed that nurses would improve the standard and continuity of patient care by sharing information through record-writing. This notion was in response to the influences of the American health care system which, in the 1970s, had adopted the idea of the nursing process as a result of discontent with nursing as a profession (De la Cuesta, 1983).

In the United Kingdom, nurses were seeking more satisfactory methods of nursing and, although diffusion of the nursing process was very rapid, it was seen as a method of improving quality of care and job satisfaction (De la Cuesta 1983).

Advantages of the nursing process are that it is patient-centred, it allows continuity and offers evidence that care is given; through which it enforces accountability (Walton 1986). By permitting evaluation it also offers a method of quality control (Robinson 1990). The process offers a measure of professional growth that allows nurses to stand alone from medicine but offers uniformity between disciplines (Renfroe *et al.* 1990). However, the nursing process is a tool and not an answer to every problem (Salvage 1985). Ultimately, what is documented reflects the character, competence and caring of the nurse (Feutz-Harter 1989).

Comprehensive care requires complete and on-going collection of data (Yura & Walsh 1988). Collecting patient information will depend on the nurse's beliefs about mankind, society, health, illness and nursing (McFarlane & Castledine 1986). Without such explicit statements of beliefs there can be little understanding of what assessment information is required (Hunt & Marks-Maran 1986; Coles & Fullenwider 1988).

Difficulties in documenting care

Owing to historical events and social pressures, the nursing process was implemented in the UK in a short period of time (De la Cuesta 1983). From the start it has been plagued by misunderstanding and misinterpretation (Walton 1986). Initially it was seen as a teaching tool rather than as a philosophy. In practice, it has been included as a framework but is not necessarily part of nurses' underlying beliefs (Miller 1985).

Tapp (1990) demonstrated that documentation was the nurse's responsibility, but it was distinctly separate, inaccurate, inconsistent and devalued in relation to caring activities. Charting was seen as a chore until it was needed for legal purposes (Gropper 1988).

Low valuation of records is an affront to the patient/client and it tends to highlight the nurses' limitations (Yura & Walsh 1988). Nurses still believe that care plans are superfluous, threatening, imposed by seniors and bear little relationship to care given (Sutcliffe 1990).

Robinson (1990) suggests that this resistance to change was due to the social climate, scant regard for the need of education and recognizing staff perceptions and needs. The result is a relentless quest for autonomy and accountability (De la Cuesta 1983).

Hays (1989) believes that paperwork is universally maligned and unsatisfactory. Record-keeping has become an overwhelming burden rather than a benefit (Morrissey-Ross 1988). The increasing complexity of recording patient information is time-consuming, and time costs money (Deane *et al.* 1986; Miller & Pastorino 1990).

Many writers note that documentation is devalued in favour of patient care when work increases (De la Cuesta 1983; Deane *et al.* 1986; Robinson 1990; Schmidt *et al.* 1990). Strategies for reducing time allocated to record-keeping without compromising quality have proved ineffective (Renfroe *et al.* 1990).

Sadly, accountability is associated with blame and control (Walsh & Ford 1990). Therefore, deviance from the plan may result in punishment or judgement of individual performance (De la Cuesta 1983). An increasing volume of nursing records are destroyed, which devalues the purpose and role of the nurse (Grier 1984).

The nursing process is said to have caused immense conflict between the ideology and reality of nursing (De la Cuesta 1983). Sutcliffe (1990) suggests that nurses hide behind paperwork to avoid patients, as the increased interaction brought about by patient-centred care increases stress and anxiety.

De la Cuesta (1983) believes that this increased anxiety is the result of the following perceptions:

(1) Documentation is seen to increase the pressure of work but, seemingly, has no obvious benefit to the patient.
(2) The nurse has an uncertain knowledge base.
(3) Talking and interviewing skills needed for data collection are not seen as working.
(4) Records are a formality designed by the bureaucracy to be completed retrospectively.

Documentation of care in the accident and emergency department

Use of the nursing process in the A/E setting is made infinitely more difficult by several factors (Walton 1986). These are recognized by Bradley (1985) as:

(1) Short stay of the patients.
(2) Variety of the presenting problems.
(3) Traditional attitude that nurses stick to rigid routines and do not have time to give individualized patient care.
(4) Strong influence of medical model.
(5) Records are time-consuming in the emergency setting and are not a priority.
(6) Planning cannot occur when it is so busy.

The development of the nursing record in the A/E department in the UK has taken place very recently and no comprehensive literature has yet been published. Work published in the USA has identified that A/E nurses lack a unique identity so there is no reason to have separate nursing records (Novotny-Dinsdale 1985; Larson 1986).

The problem as it stands is that nursing care as a theory-based subject is neither important nor valued. Therefore, nurses feel powerless and lack confidence in their role (Fox-Ungar *et al.* 1989).

Monger & Wachsmuth (1986) agree with the notion that charting in A/E appears to lack structure and was perceived as time-consuming. Therefore, charting tends to be neglected, particularly in regard to the less seriously ill or injured patients (Monger & Wachsmuth 1986; Ruth 1986).

Improving documentation

The literature suggests that improving documentation can be approached in four ways:

(1) Using a nursing assessment tool.
(2) Change.
(3) Education.
(4) Evaluation.

Using a nursing assessment tool

Professional care requires a functional health assessment as its focus (O'Neil Corrigan 1986). This would include the consideration of physical psychological and social needs, nursing diagnosis, expected outcome, the development of intervention to reduce, eliminate or prevent health problems and an evaluation of response (Calley & Siler 1987).

The nursing framework that has been used extensively in the A/E setting is that of the problem-orientated nursing record, commonly known as the SOAPE model (Gawlinski & Rasmussen 1984; Lampe 1985; Coles & Full-enwider 1988; Grieve 1988; Bracy & Wicikowski 1989; Hays 1989). This was adapted for nursing by Cormack (1980) and is described in Table 8.1. This model captures the essence of professional decision making and can be adapted to incorporate a nursing rather than a medical model, at the same time complementing independent and interdependent roles of the nurse in the A/E department (Fox-Ungar *et al.* 1989).

Gawlinski & Rasmussen (1984) and Bracey & Wicikowski (1989) suggest that the advantage of using this model are as follows:

(1) Patient-centred.
(2) Uses problem-solving process.
(3) Common language between disciplines.
(4) Improves communication, trust and confidence of staff.
(5) Increases efficiency.
(6) Evaluates effectiveness/quality of care.
(7) Has explicit implications for research or service evaluation.
(8) Easy to read and quick to write, so paperwork can be kept to a minimum.

Table 8.1 Interpretation of SOAPE model (Cormack 1980; reproduced by kind permission of *Nursing Times* where this paper first appeared on 3 April 1980, **76**:9, 37).

S – Subjective evidence of the problem (what the patient says or complains of).
O – Objective evidence of the problem (what the nurse observes in relation to the problem).
A – Assessment of the problem (nursing diagnosis).
P – Plan of nursing intervention (diagnostic, therapeutic, advice/explanation).
E – Expected/actual outcome of nursing intervention (allows for evaluation of nursing care).

Coles & Fullenwider (1988) suggest that disadvantages of inconsistency and increased writing time reduce morale. However, Monger & Wachsmuth (1986) and Edelstein (1990) argue that these disadvantages are outweighed by advantages and can be overcome by consideration of the change process and education of staff.

Change

Overcoming problems of documenting care requires use of a change theory to convert concept into reality (Murphy *et al.* 1988). Discussion of proposed changes allows staff to develop ownership of records, ensuring that they are more likely to be used (Noone 1987; Walker 1990). The involvement allows everybody to explore new ideas so that they are able to see the new developments and trends (Monger & Wachsmuth 1986).

Team-work is essential to allow staff control of their own practice (Sovie 1989). Improving communication and documentation requires time, leadership, reflection and discussion (Edelstein 1990). Nurses need a favourable environment and adequate support in order to explore their own attitudes and beliefs about record-keeping (Kitson 1986; Renfroe *et al.* 1990; Edelstein 1990).

Lewin's change theory of 'unfreezing–moving– refreezing' has been used in the introduction of new documentation (Gawlinski & Rasmussen 1984; Monger & Wachsmuth 1986). Noone (1987) preferred Lippett's theory of planned change. Walker (1990) advocates gradual introduction of change and willingness by the change agent to show trust and provide future support. Change must be seen as dynamic and on-going (Halm 1990).

Whether a change theory is used or not, the challenge lies in completing records that are simple, understandable, cost-effective and efficient, and which enable the monitoring of quality (Decker 1985; Weeks & Darrah 1985; Yura & Walsh 1988).

Education

Education is required to support change (De la Cuesta 1983). Nurses need to be assisted in the identification of a body of nursing knowledge (Grier 1984). They need the opportunity to explore their own beliefs about nursing as a profession, to discuss the importance of documentation and to practise recording care according to a systematic agreed framework that reflects their beliefs (Yura & Walsh 1988).

Writing skills need to involve organization, relationships, nursing activities, patient outcomes, critical thinking and decision making (Lampe 1989). Directing this learning involves teaching, promotion of change and increased accountability (Edelstein 1990).

Evaluation

One of the most mismanaged stages of the nursing process is evaluation (Hunt & Marks-Maran 1986). Bergman (1982) suggests that evaluation should reveal strengths and weaknesses and ultimately benefits all those involved.

Concerns about quality and standard setting have been expressed for years but it is clear that all areas should have effective measures for quality (Hunt 1987). Nurses should strive for efficiency and effectiveness in the delivery of care (Nadzam 1987, Rowden 1990).

Evaluation of nursing care involves creativity, self-assessment and peer review (Donabedian 1969). It depends on the motivation of the leader in acting and involving others and in offering constructive criticism (Kitson

1986). Measures of evaluation do not have to be rigid (Lorentzon 1987). Measurement tools need to be developed to suit an area and may result in better care, better use of resources and greater satisfaction for nurses (Mackie & Welch 1982).

One method of evaluation is retrospective chart audit which involves systematic inspection of an agreed percentage of discharged patient records (Pearson 1991). Audit asks the question, 'Has good care been given?' (Craig 1987).

Wandelt & Ager (1974) argue that a great deal of care is never written down at all so auditing can never be complete. However, others have found auditing helpful in improving record writing, professional practice, communication and staff morale (Phaneuf 1976; Ellson 1984; Novotny-Dinsdale 1985; Yura & Walsh 1988; Halm 1990; Orr & Bryant 1990; Walker 1990).

Audit

Phaneuf (1976) developed an audit that involves self-regulation in nursing practice. The audit is retrospective, easy, economical and provides a good global perspective (Willis & Linwood 1984). Phaneuf (1976) suggests that comparative audits using problem-orientated and traditional records might assist in deciding whether problem-orientated recording reflects improvements in quality of care.

In summary, the aim of documentation is to facilitate communication of individual care, to provide continuity, to act as a mechanism for accountability and to provide a legal record of care, a potential measure of quality and a method of expanding the scientific body of nursing knowledge (WHO 1983).

Record-writing is a particular problem in the A/E department where influence of the medical model, rigid routines and short stay of patients with a variety of different problems make planning and documentation of care very difficult. The literature suggests that most of the evidence supporting changes to record keeping in A/E settings are based on descriptive reports rather than on empirical research. It is curiosity and need for scientific evidence that provide the impetus for this study.

The study

The aim of this study was to evaluate the effect of introducing a nursing record using the SOAPE model in the A/E department and preparing the staff to use it. This hypothesis follows: 'The use of the SOAPE problem-orientated record will be associated with an improvement in the documentation of care and, in turn, the quality of care'.

These criteria were selected for the following reasons:

(1) The Phaneuf audit tool exists to measure the quality of documentation and has been widely used, and tested for validity and reliability (Phaneuf 1976; Ventura *et al.* 1986; Manfredi 1986; Pearson 1991).
(2) Conditions leading to good documentation also lead to good nursing care (Phaneuf 1976).
(3) Previous studies concerning documentation provide suggestions on study design (Ruth 1986; Weeks & Darrah 1985; Walker 1990; Deane *et al.* 1986; Gawlinski & Rasmussen 1984; Monger & Wachsmuth 1986).
(4) Documentation is a legal requirement and a mechanism for account-ability; therefore, records need to reflect care given (WHO 1983).

Method

The research setting was an accident and emergency department in central London, England. The department is divided into a variety of clinical areas: triage, box, waiting area, cubicles, dressings, theatre and resuscitation rooms. The department is open 24 hours a day and, at the time of the study, received 70 000 patients per year.

The patient population included adults of both sexes and varying ages; 11% of those presenting for care were children. Owing to the geographical position of this department there tended to be a high transient population of commuters and tourists, plus those residents and homeless presenting with problems associated with the unavoidable stresses of inner-city life.

At the time of this study the nursing staff numbered 50 and included seven sisters, 10 senior staff nurses, 21 staff nurses, two enrolled nurses and 10 student nurses. They were managed by a senior nurse. All staff, except the senior nurse and two sisters, worked internal rotation to night duty. Two medical consultants were responsible for the department, one of whom was always present or on call. They had the support of a senior registrar. Day-to-day medical decisions were made by a team of senior house officers who worked a shift system. Other permanent staff included the lecturer practi-tioner who was responsible for education/service liaison, a team of recep-tionists and two secretaries.

The organization of care varied between task allocation and patient allocation, depending on the member of staff involved. Documentation of nursing care was carried out on a nursing record for all patients in the cubicles and resuscitation rooms. Patients in the waiting area had their assessment written on the medical notes.

This area was selected for exploration in response to problems identified with record writing and as a result of auditing the learning environment.

Evaluation approach

The study adopted an evaluation approach. The time frame in Fig. 8.1 illustrates the process followed. Consent was obtained from the senior nurse manager and consultants, as patient records were to be reviewed. Permission from the ethical committee was not deemed necessary as documentation of care is a legal responsibility of the nurse and should be part of everyday practice (WHO 1983).

A working party of nursing staff identified that difficulties in documenting records were due to:

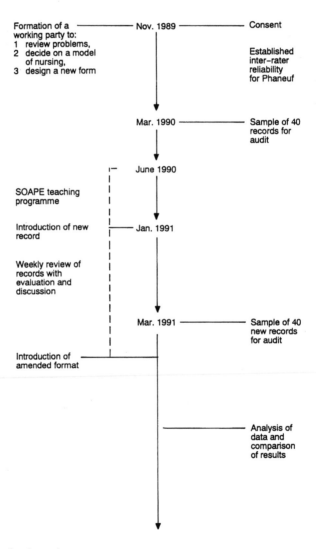

Fig. 8.1   The timeframe for the study.

(1) Lack of understanding of why records were important.
(2) Use of a nursing record which did not allow documentation of continuity of care and offered no framework for assessment

Models of nursing were discussed at great length but it was felt that they were too detailed to use in the emergency setting. Following an extensive literature review and weekly meetings, we agreed to use the SOAPE model.

The new form (Fig. 8.2) was designed and ordered in December 1990. Owing to the holiday period and nature of the bureaucracy, the forms did not arrive until February 1991.

Phaneuf's audit tool

Phaneuf's nursing audit tool was chosen as an instrument for the following reasons, previously identified by Willis & Linwood (1984) and supported by Pearson (1991):

(1) It responds to the management need for the attainment of quality and the legal requirements of accountability towards patient, profession and public.
(2) It is economical in use of time, cost and personnel required, in comparison to other methods.
(3) It allows for on-going corrective active or formative evaluation so feedback can be immediate.
(4) It has been tried and tested in a variety of clinical and community settings.
(5) It gives those nurses a sense of achievement when they feel that they have been instrumental in improving standards of care.

In addition, it has been tested for reliability and validity (Ventura *et al.* 1986; Manfredi 1986).

Phaneuf's audit schedule is nursing-process-orientated. It is based on seven functions of nursing (Table 8.2), which are divided into 50 components and given scores accordingly. Each function can be assigned a range, so that it can be analysed individually (Phaneuf 1976). Inter-rater reliability is achieved by trial audits to establish majority agreement (Phaneuf 1976). Unanimity in judgement is not required on each of 50 items; however, there should be agreement as to the quality of the execution of each nursing function (Phaneuf 1976).

Sample

The sample chosen was influenced by constraints of time and number of auditors available. It was decided that 40 pre-audit and 40 post-audit records

ACCIDENT and EMERGENCY PATIENT CARE RECORD

A/E no: .... Hospital no: ....
Surname: .... Age: ....
First names: .... DoB: ....

Date: ....
Time of arrival: ....
Time of assessment: ....
Triaged by: ....

Last attendance: ....
Mode of arrival: ....
Brought in from: ....
Accompanied by: ....

SUBJECTIVE

HPI:

PMH: Medication:

Social history:

OBJECTIVE

ASSESSMENT:

PLAN: Diagnostic   Therapeutic   Advice/explanation

PROGRESS NOTES

TIME	OBSERVATIONS	SIGN

OUTCOME: Δ:

Fig. 8.2 Example of the new form.

Table 8.2 The seven functions of Phaneuf's nursing audit (reproduced from Nursing Audit Chart Review Schedule (Phaneuf 1976), Appleton & Lange, Norwalk, Connecticut).

I	Application and execution of physician's legal orders
II	Observations of symptoms and reactions
III	Supervision of the patient
IV	Supervision of those participating in care (except physician)
V	Reporting and recording
VI	Application and execution of nursing procedures and techniques
VII	Promotion of physical and emotional health by direction and teaching

could be managed for this study. The records were selected randomly from patients presenting with the problems of chest pain, head injury, excessive menstrual bleeding and drug overdose. This is an example of purposive sampling (Polit & Hungler 1987).

Teaching programme

The teaching programme included four sessions run twice a week. On completion of the sessions the staff would be able to:

(1) Identify the components of the SOAPE model (session 1).
(2) Assess the patient's needs using the subjective–objective format (session 2).
(3) Plan care giving clear directions that could be followed by others (session 3).
(4) Complete a new patient care record for an individual attending the A/E department, demonstrating progress notes and continuity of care, and discuss the advantages and difficulties experienced (session 4).

The aim was to move the staff towards the internalization stage of the experiential taxonomy (Kenworthy & Micklin 1989).

Once the new record was introduced, review and discussion of the records was held weekly with the staff on duty. This acted as formative evaluation (Phaneuf 1976).

Limitations and assumptions

Limitations

The limitations of the study are as follows:

(1) Small sample, matched for patient problem only and did not include age, sex, time of presentation to A/E and nurse attending to the problem.
(2) Data were limited to a one-month period.

(3) Documentation may not reflect care given, i.e. all care given is not written (Wandelt & Ager 1974).
(4) Hawthorne effect – knowledge of being included may be sufficient to cause people to change their behaviour (Polit & Hungler 1987).
(5) Same person is implementing and evaluating this research.
(6) Results will be limited to one A/E setting.

Assumptions

The assumptions of the study are as follows:

(1) Phaneuf is a reliable and valid instrument for measuring quality of care.
(2) Phaneuf is valid and reliable for use in A/E setting.
(3) Staff that completed the sample of new records had completed the teaching programme.

Results

The mean of total and functions scores were calculated for each sample and plotted on the quality profile line graph (Phaneuf 1976) (Fig. 8.3).

Comparison of the total mean score showed that the overall quality of care had risen from poor to incomplete. Function I had risen to a level of good. Function II remained in the incomplete category. Functions III and V had risen to incomplete. Function VI had risen to excellent. Functions IV and VII

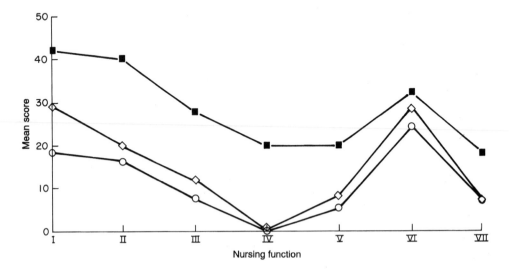

Fig. 8.3 Quality profile line graph. —■—, maximum score; —◇—, post March 1991; —○—, pre March 1990.

showed no change. The number of charts in each scoring range is tabled in Fig. 8.4. Overall, the unsafe and poor categories decreased and incomplete, good and excellent categories increased.

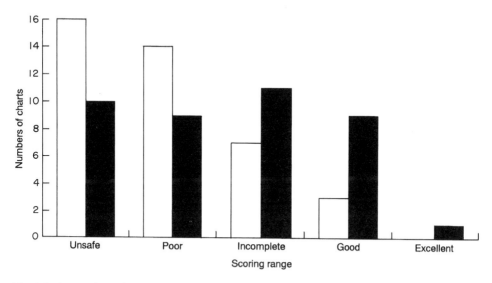

Fig. 8.4 Comparison of the number of charts from each scoring range. □, March 1990; ■, March 1991.

A chi-square distribution was calculated for each of the nursing functions (Table 8.3). This showed that the post-audit scores (Y) were significantly higher, in functions I, II, III, V, VI, than the pre-audit scores (X), using a one-tailed test. Post-audit scores in functions IV and VII were not significantly higher.

As such difficulties had been experienced establishing inter-rater reliability, the kappa statistic (k) was established for each component. When there

Table 8.3 The chi-square for total score and the nursing function score.

Function	χ^2	d.f.	$P \leqslant 0.05$ one-tailed
Total	7.12	3	Sig.
I	7.04	3	Sig.
II	6.41	3	Sig.
III	8.32	3	Sig.
IV	0	1	Not sig.
V	13.6	3	Sig.
VI	0.13	2	Sig.
VII	0.32	3	Not sig.

Sig. = significant.

is total agreement then k = 1 (Siegal & Castellan 1988). The function means of k ranged between 0.56 and 0.77 (Table 8.4). A percentage agreement was calculated for the six components that did not demonstrate significant agreement. The results ranged from 90% to 97.5%.

Table 8.4 The mean and range of k for each function.

Function	Mean of k	Range
I	0.77	0.72–0.83
II	0.56	0.16–0.75
III	0.7	0.46–1
IV	Complete agreement	
V	0.67	0.43–1
VI	0.63	0.02–0.87
VII	0.59	0.04–1

Discussion

The results have shown that the introduction of this model in this A/E department has made significant improvement to practice. So the hypothesis can be supported. There are several possible explanations for the results, which relate to each function, the approach, inter-rater reliability, the sample and the teaching programme used in this study.

There was significant improvement in application and execution of medical orders. The charts allowed for medical diagnosis to be completed but also nurses were encouraged to document progress which often included waiting for doctors' orders or decisions. It is not certain whether the improvement was due to the model, the format of the record or increased staff awareness.

Observations of symptoms and reactions had significantly improved, but remained in the same scoring range. Observations of physical function were always a priority but were often taken without discrimination. However, observations of feelings were not always documented and staff reported in the formative evaluation sessions that they found feelings difficult to record.

Supervision of the patient was significantly improved. Again, it was difficult to be sure if this had been due to the model or the layout of the record; however, problems were identified and continuity of care monitored. Safety of the patient was difficult to assess as this would not necessarily be recorded on each individual chart. Assumptions were made that if a patient was allocated to an area then specific emergency equipment would be available. Care planning and goal setting which were required to identify patient adaptation was clearly an area of weakness. The staff argued that this was because there is little time to plan care as their action has to be immediate. This may be an area for further work in the future.

Supervision of those participating in care showed no significant improvement. There were one or two problems with this section which had previously been identified by Manfredi (1986). First, supervision of other nurses would not be written on the patient record and therefore was disregarded. Second, the patient groups chosen would not necessarily be expected to participate in care at this stage, due to their unstable or unresponsive condition. Also, family would often not be present during initial emergency care. The raters were forced to select the 'no' option, reducing the overall rating. A 'not applicable' option may have been more appropriate.

Recording and reporting of care showed a significant improvement. Reporting essential facts to the physician was assumed if continuing care was recorded, as the medical staff constantly referred to the patient care records.

It was interesting that 'continuity', documented most frequently, referred to what the doctor was doing rather than an evaluation of patient progress. This was addressed in the formative sessions.

Application and execution of nursing procedures and techniques (function VI) showed a significant improvement and scored in the highest range. However, most of the components were 'not applicable'. It was very task-orientated so points were only scored if the procedure related to the assessment of patient needs.

Promotion of physical and emotional health by direction and teaching (function VII) showed no significant improvement in quality. Much teaching and promotion of health was said to go on in practice but was not seen as something to document. This may be a good example of the need for an observation tool to be used in conjunction with the audit so that actual practice may be measured.

Problems

The difficulties experienced using evaluation research were in relation to gaining staff co-operation and commitment. Although the working party met at regular intervals, the membership changed completely during the period of the study. The timing changed slightly as the new records took longer to arrive than expected. The order then ran out before the next arrived so temporarily the staff had to revert to using the old record.

One of the weaknesses of this study is that it was initiated, implemented and evaluated by the researcher. Also, evaluation research is not a scientific, controlled method (Polit & Hungler 1987). Some would argue that audit alone cannot measure quality of care. However, Phaneuf (1976) believes that record audit reveals commendable strengths and weaknesses that can be corrected; in all, it raises awareness.

Manfredi (1986) argues that the Phaneuf audit tool appeared inappropriate for short-stay patients as detailed records were not necessary. However, this study revealed that records which scored highly were not necessarily lengthy; it was the quality of information recorded that was important.

During the data-collection stage the raters had difficulty in using the tool for several reasons. First, this tool was designed for use in the USA which has a very different culture from that of the UK. This made for laborious interpretation of the jargon for use in relation to British nursing practice. Secondly, Phaneuf (1976) suggests that the functions reflect the nursing process, but they were more like roles of the nurse. Third nursing assessment should be the first priority for patient care and also for record writing, giving information to the patient/family or communicating with nurses in other areas. Medical orders should influence the plan of care and medical diagnosis should be included in the outcome.

As Manfredi (1986) noted, it is uncertain whether doctors' orders should be included in nursing audit, because when the doctor fails to fulfil his/her responsibilities or is unable to make a diagnosis, the overall rating of nursing care is lowered. In a multidisciplinary setting, where roles of doctor and nurse depend on each other, medical care cannot be ignored. Perhaps there is a need for a multidisciplinary record and audit in the future.

Scoring

Raters found that scoring for the audit was not based on obvious principles. The weighting applied suggested that the underlying philosophy was medically oriented, not based on a nursing model. Phaneuf (1976) argues that functions I–V are essential for safe nursing practice; however, it was felt that all patients should also be rated in forms of promotion of physical and emotional health and consideration of continuing care, whether this was provided at home or in hospital.

Overall, raters found that the retrospective audit of nursing notes could be done at a convenient time so that it did not detract from clinical practice. Looking at documentation reflects the actions of all those involved and demonstrates the organizational method of care. As raters became more adept at auditing, awareness about their own care and record writing was enhanced, resulting in change of practice.

Although the scoring alone had little meaning, the graphs of comparative results clearly showed areas of strength and weakness and have provided incentive for further improvement of practice. The sample was small in relation to total population and was not representative of all patients presenting for care. If documentation of care is a legal responsibility, all patients must have nursing records and a sample for audit should be selected from the whole population, regardless of presenting problem.

It was almost impossible to match nurses from March 1990 to March 1991. This was partly because nurses had not signed their notes. A large proportion of the staff had moved onto other posts during this period.

It is unlikely that quality of documentation improved due to the teaching programme alone. First, the change in method of documentation naturally altered the nurses' writing style. Second, the teaching only addressed reasons for documenting care, the meaning of the model and a brief introduction to writing skills. The remaining problems and uncertainties were tackled through formative evaluation sessions. They were kept flexible and informal as the sessions were frequently interrupted by emergencies.

Third, not all 40 members of staff attended all the sessions. Ten completed session four and happily tried out the new record and offered examples for discussion. Another 20 completed session three. The others only attended the introductory session, due to holiday, night duty, study leave and personal choice. Some clearly did not like the teaching style and found it very threatening to explore the nature of their own practice. It may have been ambitious to expect all the staff to achieve internalization.

Nursing implications

The study has highlighted a number of issues relating to the professional responsibilities of the nurse. In A/E work nurses need to identify their unique role, which combines medical skills with nursing expertise.

Despite limitations of this study the process of evaluation has allowed staff to participate in and achieve a change in practice which they needed to believe possible. It has also allowed medical staff to consider the nurse's role and responsibilities as an interdependent practitioner. The study has contributed towards removing myths about the nursing process and models of nursing that staff considered time-consuming and distracting. It has offered documentary evidence that accountability can be maintained through short concise notes, which reflect continuity of care.

Conclusion

This study produced results that provide an incentive to extend nursing audit in the future. There was significant improvement in documentation of care in the A/E department during the period of this study. It is not clear whether this was due to the model or the teaching session, as both were dependent on each other. However, the model helped to give nurses a framework on which to base care and teach others. It also allowed flexibility for assessment of individual needs. This experience gave the researcher an opportunity to carry out evaluation research in practice and the desire to look critically at other quality assurance measures in the future.

Although the study was small and limited to one department it is hoped that the ideas explored will give incentive to those working in other A/E departments.

Recommendations

If quality in practice is to be maintained, formative evaluation sessions need to continue. It is suggested that audit is performed at monthly intervals, using a probability sample of 10% of the population; this would require a committee of interested staff to learn about the Phaneuf audit tool and to set goals for future improvements in practice. Difficulties in reaching consensus may be overcome by auditing together (Phaneuf 1976). Alternative quality measures also need to be considered in order to ensure that what is documented is actually carried out.

Further teaching is needed, particularly in relation to planning care, health education and discharge planning. Sessions could also include professional issues, for example, accountability and alternative quality measures. Staff should be encouraged to document care as well as medical interventions.

The headings used on the record need to be altered to incorporate everyday language that can be interpreted and taught to new staff in the A/E department.

Further studies need to be carried out in other A/E departments, before generalizations could be made regarding applicability of this model elsewhere. It may be that further work could allow for the development and testing of alternative instruments for measuring quality of care in the A/E setting. Collaborative, multidisciplinary records and audit need to be developed and explored.

Postscript

Since this study was completed, formative evaluations have continued and the new record has been amended to incorporate clearer terminology. Results of the study were shared with the staff, and one of the sisters has shown interest in forming a new working party of nurses willing to learn the Phaneuf audit tool.

This demonstrates that a record audit alone can provide incentive for A/E nurses to become involved in evaluation of their own practice; and that self-determination, collaboration and evaluation are the way forward.

Acknowledgements

I would like to thank all the staff from the Accident and Emergency Department at University College Hospital, London, for that participation, support and commitment. Without their help this study would not have been feasible.

I would also like to thank Mrs K. Manley for her supervision, advice and encouragement, Miss J. Clarke for her commitment and support in mastering the audit tool and Miss A. Townley for her reliability and patience in typing the final dissertation.

References

Bergman, R. (1982) Evaluation of nursing care: could it make a difference? *International Journal of Nursing Studies*, **19**(2), 53–60.

Bracey, R. & Wicikowski, D. (1989) Apportioning care. *Nursing Times*, **85**(19), 49–51.

Bradley, D. (1985) Adapting the process. *Nursing Times*, **81**(23), 38–40.

Calley, I.S. & Siler, P.V. (1987) Nursing process: a framework for documentation. *Emphasis: Nursing*, **2**(2), 84–91.

Coles, M.C. & Fullenwider, S.D. (1988) Documentation managing the dilemma. *Nursing Management*, **19**(2), 65–6, 70, 72.

Cormack, D.F.S. (1980) The nursing process: an application of the SOAPE model. *Nursing Times, Occasional paper*, **76**(9), 37–9.

Costello, S. & Summers, B.Y. (1985) Documenting patient care: getting it all together. *Nursing Management*, **16**(6), 31–2, 34.

Cowan, V. (1987) Documentation. *Nursing*, **14**, 527–9.

Craig, D. (1987) Audit design. *Recent Advances in Nursing*, **17**, 65–93.

Deane, D., McElroy, M.H. & Alden, S. (1986) Documentation: meeting requirements while maximising productivity. *Nursing Economics*, **4**(4), 174–8.

Decker, G.H. (1985) Quality assurance: accent on monitoring. *Nursing Management*, **16**(11), 20–22, 24.

De la Cuesta, C. (1983) The nursing process: from development to implementation. *Journal of Advanced Nursing*, **8**(5), 365–71.

Donabedian, A. (1969) Some issues in evaluating the quality of nursing care. *American Journal of Public Health*, **59**, 1833–6.

Edelstein, J. (1990) A study of nursing documentation. *Nursing Management*, **21**(11), 40–43, 46.

Ellson, S.K. (1984) It can improve your patient records. *The Journal of Continuing Education in Nursing*, **15**(3), 78–81.

Feutz-Harter, S. (1989) Legal insights: documentation principles and pitfalls. *JONA*, **19**(12), 7–9.

Fox-Ungar, E., Newell, G. & Guilbault, K. (1989) Documentation: communicating professionalism. *Nursing Management*, **20**(1), 65–66, 68, 70.

Gay, P. (1983) Get it in writing. *Nursing Management*, **14**(3), 32–5.

Gawlinski, A. & Rasmussen, S. (1984) Improving documentation through use of change theory. *Focus on Critical Care*, **15**(3), 78–81.

Grier, M.R. (1984) Information processing in nursing practice. *Annual Review of Nursing Research*, **2**, 265–87.

Grieve, G.P. (1988) Clinical examination and the SOAP mnemonic. *Physiotherapy*, **74**(2), 97.

Gropper, E. (1988) Does your charting reflect your worth? *Geriatric Nursing*, Mar/Apr, 99–101.

Halm, M.A. (1990) Developing a unit-based quality assurance tool. *Journal of Nursing Quality Assurance*, **4**(2), 18–27.

Harris, R.B. (1979) A strong vote for nursing process. *American Journal of Nursing*, **79**, 1999–2001.

Hays, J.C. (1989) Voices in the record. *Image: Journal of Nursing Scholarship*, **21**(4), 200–204.

Hershey, N. & Lawrence, R. (1986) The influence of charting upon liability determination. *Journal of Nursing Administration*, Mar/April, 35–7.

Hunt, J. (1987) Assuring quality. *Nursing Times*, **83**(44), 29–31.

Hunt, J. & Marks-Maran, D. (1986) *Nursing Care Plans*. John Wiley, Chichester.

Kenworthy, N. & Nicklin, P.J. (1989) *Teaching and Assessing in Nursing Practice*. Scutari Press, London.

Kitson, A.L. (1966) Taking action. *Nursing Times*, **82**(36), 52–4.

Lampe, S.S. (1985) Focus charting: streamlining documentation. *Nursing Management*, **16**(7), 43–6.

Lampe, S.S. (1989) Nursing documentation: a new perspective. *JONA*, **19**(3), 3.

Larson, L. (1986) Nursing diagnosis: defining it and fitting it into the nursing process. *Journal of Emergency Nursing*, **12**(3), 127–8.

Lorentzon, M. (1987) Quality in nursing: the state of the art. *Senior Nurse*, **7**(6), 11–12.

McFarlane, J.K. & Castledine, G. (1986) *A Guide to the Practice of Nursing Using the Nursing Process*. C.V. Mosby, London.

Mackie, L.C.R. & Welch, J.W. (1982) Quality assurance audit for the nursing process. *Nursing Times*, **77**(43), 1757–8.

Manfredi, C. (1986) Reliability and validity of the Phaneuf nursing audit. *Western Journal of Nursing Research*, **8**(2), 168–80.

Miller, A. (1985) Are you using the nursing process? *Nursing Times*, **85**(50), 36.

Miller, P. & Pastorino, C. (1990) Daily nursing documentation can be quick and thorough! *Nursing Management*, **21**(11), 47–9.

Monger, M. & Wachsmuth, C. (1986) An ED nursing documentation tool and the process of planned change. *Journal of Emergency Nursing*, **12**(6), 370–77.

Morgan, E. (1985) New chart forms solve old problems. *American Journal of Nursing*, **85**, 93–5.

Morrissey-Ross, M. (1988) Documentation: if you haven't written it, you haven't done it. *Nursing Clinics of North America*, **23**(2), 363–71.

Murphy, J., Begilinger, J.E. & Johnson, B. (1988) Charting by exception: meeting the challenge of cost containment. *Nursing Management*, **19**(2), 56–72.

Nadzam, D.M. (1987) Documentation evaluation system: streamlining quality of care and personnel evaluations. *Nursing Management*, **18**(11), 38–42.

Noone, J. (1987) Planned change: putting theory into practice. *Clinical Nurse Specialist*, **1**(1), 25–9.

Novotny-Dinsdale, V. (1985) Implementation of nursing diagnosis in one emergency department. *Journal of Emergency Nursing*, **11**(3), 140–44.

O'Neill Corrigan, J. (1986) Functional health pattern assessment in the emergency department. *Journal of Emergency Nursing*, **12**(3), 163–7.

Orr, I. & Bryant, R. (1990) Development of an audit system. *Senior Nurse*, **10**(9), 14–15.

Pearson, A. (ed.) *Nursing Quality Measurement: Quality Assurance Methods for Peer Review*. John Wiley & Sons, Chichester.

Phaneuf, M.C. (1976) *The Nursing Audit – Self Regulation in Practice*, 2nd edn. Appleton Century Crofts, New York.

Polit, D.F. & Hungler, B.P. (1987) *Nursing Research: Principles and Methods*, 3rd edn. Lippincott, Philadelphia

Renfroe, D.H., O'Sullivan, P.S. & McGee, G.W. (1990) The relationship of attitude, subjective norm and behavioural intent to documentation behaviour of nurses. *Scholarly Inquiry for Nursing Practice: An International Journal*, **4**(1), 47–60.

Robinson, D. (1990) Two decades of 'the process'. *Senior Nurse*, **10**(2), 4–6.

Rowden, R. (1990) Quality of care. *Nursing Times*, **86**(8), 29–30.

Ruth, J.P. (1986) Nursing diagnosis in the emergency department. *Journal of Emergency Nursing*, **12**(6), 310–13.

Salvage, J. (1985) *The Politics of Nursing*. Heinemann, London.

Schmidt, D., Gathers, B., Stewart, M., Tyler, C., Hawkins, M. & Denton, K. (1990) Charting for accountability. *Nursing Management*, **21**(11), 50–52.

Siegal, S. & Castellan, N.J. (1988) *Non Parametric Statistics for the Behavioural Sciences*, 2nd edn. McGraw Hill, New York.

Sklar, C. (1984) The patient's record, an invaluable communication tool. *Canadian Nurse*, **80**(5), 50, 52.

Sovie, M.D. (1989) Clinical nursing practices and patient outcomes: evaluation, evolution and revolution. *Nursing Economics*, **7**(2), 79–85.

Sutcliffe, E. (1990) Reviewing the process progress. *Senior Nurse*, **10**(9), 9–13.

Tapp, R.A. (1990) Inhibitors and facilitators to the documentation of nursing practice. *Western Journal of Nursing Research*, **12**(2), 229–40.

Vasey, E.K. (1979) Writing your patient's care plan efficiently. *Nursing*, **9**(4), 67–71.

Ventura, M., Hageman, P., Slakter, M. & Fox, R. (1986) Interrater reliabilities for two measures of nursing care quality. *Research in Nursing and Health*, **3**, 25–32.

Walker, C. (1990) Introducing new forms: over-coming resistance. *Journal of Nursing Quality Assurance*, **4**(2), 82–5.

Walsh, M. & Ford, P. (1990) *Nursing Rituals: Research and Rational Actions*. Heinemann, Oxford.

Walton, I. (1986) *The Nursing Process in Perspective: A Literature Review*. University of York. DHSS, London.

Wandelt, M.A. & Ager, J.W. (1974) *Quality Patient Care Scale*. Appleton-Century-Crofts, New York.

Weeks, L.C. & Darrah, P. (1985) The documentation dilemma: a practical solution. *JONA*, **15**(11), 22–7.

Willis, L.D. & Linwood, M.E. (eds) (1984) *Measuring the Quality of Care*, Churchill Livingstone, Edinburgh.

World Health Organization (1983) *Documentation of the Nursing Process: Report on a Working Group*, 8–12 Dec 1980, Berne. WHO Regional Office for Europe.

Yura, H. & Walsh, M.B. (1988) *The Nursing Process*, 5th edn. Appleton & Lange, Norwalk, Connecticut.

Further reading

Blansfield, J., Fackler, C. & Bergeron, K. (1985) Developing standardized care plans: one emergency department's experience. *Journal of Emergency Nursing*, **11**(6), 304–309.

Chalmers, H.A. (1989) Theories and models of nursing and nursing process. *Recent Advances in Nursing*, **24**, 32–46.

Chavasse, J. (1987) A comparison of three modes of nursing. *Nurse Education Today*, **7**(4), 177–86.

Christensen, M.H. (1990) Peer auditing. *Nursing Management*, **21**(1), 50–52.

Cline, A. (1989) Streamlined documentation through exceptional charting. *Nursing Management*, **20**(2), 62–4.

Distefano, J. (1984) ED nursing process notes. *Journal of Emergency Nursing*, **10**(4), 225–6.

Hadfield, L. (1989) In search of excellence in accident and emergency. *Nursing Standard*, **25**(3), 19–22.

Henderson, V. (1987) The nursing process in perspective. *Journal of Advanced Nursing*, **12**(6), 657–8.

Hinkle, D.E., Wiersma, W. & Jurs, S.G. (1982) *Basic Behavioural Statistics*, Houghton Mifflin, Boston.

Kilpack, V. & Dobson-Brassard, S. (1987) Intershift report: oral communication using the nursing process. *Journal of Neuroscience Nursing*, **19**(5), 266–70.

Leavell, H.R. & Clark, E.G. (1965) *Preventive Medicine for the Doctor in his Community – an Epidemiologic Approach*, 3rd edn. McGraw-Hill, New York.

Lesnik, M.H. & Anderson, B.E. (1955) *Nursing Practice and the Law*, 2nd edn. Lippincott, Philadelphia.

McPhee, A. (1987) Teaching students how to chart. *Nurse Educator*, **12**(4), 33–6.

Montemuro, M. (1988) Core documentation: a complete system for charting nursing care. *Nursing Management*, **19**(1), 28–32.

Openshaw, S. (1984) Literature review: measurements of adequate care. *International Journal of Nursing Studies*, **21**(4), 295–304.

Owen, L., Bojanowski, C. & Vermillion, C. (1988) A process to improve the documentation of nurse's notes. *Journal of Nursing Staff Development*, Summer, 104–11.

Peterson, C. (1985) Cut your paperwork with this 4 minute ED admission form. *Nursing*, Feb, 56–7.

Posey, V.M. & Howell, J.S. (1984) A timesaving flow sheet for life threatening emergencies. *Nursing*, May 8–9.

Richards, D.A. & Lambert, P. (1987) The nursing process: the effects on patient's satisfaction with nursing care. *Journal of Advanced Nursing*, **12**(5), 559–62.

Robinson, J. (ed.) (1978) *Documenting Patient Care Responsibly: Nursing Skill Book*. Intermed Communications, Horsham, Pennsylvania.

Royal College of Nursing (1990) *Promoting Professional Excellence*. RCN, London.

Schön, D. (1983) *Educating the Reflective Practitioner. Toward a New Design for Teaching and Learning*. Jossey-Bass, San Francisco.

Smeltzer, C. & Hinshaw, A.S. (1988) Research: clinical integration for excellent patient care. *Nursing Management*, **19**(1), 38–40.

Steinaker, M.W. & Bell, M.R. (1979) *The Experiential Taxonomy*. Academic Press, New York.

Townson, D. (1985) Form and function: marry the two. *Nursing Success Today*, **2**(5), 37–9.

United Kingdom Central Council (1984) *Code of Professional Conduct for the Nurse, Midwife and Health Visitor*, 2nd edn. UKCC, London.

Vogt, J., Miesle, A., Dreier, R. & Aubry, A.(1985) Flex – primary care delivery and communications system. *Journal of Emergency Nursing*, **11**(2), 85–90.

Weed, L. (1971) *Preparing and Maintaining the Problem-Orientated Record: The Promis Method*. The Press of Case, Western Reserve University.

Whelan, J. (1991) Troublespots in quality assurance. *Nursing Standard*, **5**(25), 36–8.

White, R. (1980) *Educating for Clinical Excellence*. Twenty Eighth Annual Oration. The New South Wales College of Nursing. Richards PTY Ltd.

Wilson, R.A. (1987) *Hospital Wide OA*. Saunders, Toronto.

Workgroups of European Nurse Researchers (1985) 7th Workgroup Meeting. *Nursing Research – Does it make a Difference?* Royal College of Nursing, London.

Wright, D. (1984) An introduction to the evaluation of nursing care: a review of the literature. *Journal of Advanced Nursing*, **9**(5), 457–67.

Chapter 9
Psychosocial recovery from adult liver transplantation: a literature review

STEVEN P. WAINWRIGHT, *MSc, BSc(Hons), PGCE, RGN*
Lecturer in Nursing Studies, Department of Nursing Studies, King's College,
University of London, England

Liver transplantation is now the treatment of choice for patients with end stage chronic liver disease. However, there appears to be no review of the literature on patient recovery from liver transplantation. This comprehensive review presents a picture of the state of the art in liver transplantation, and considers literature on psychiatric, functional status, and quality of life aspects of patient recovery. Numerous suggestions for further research are made.

Introduction

Liver transplantation is undoubtedly a life changing, life threatening and potentially a life ending experience. Moreover:

'Liver transplantation is now becoming routine worldwide... Hepatologists have now reached the stage of thinking of liver transplantation whenever confronted by a patient with advanced chronic liver disease' (Sherlock & Dooley 1993).

It is hoped that this comprehensive review will increase insight into the recovery of this group of patients, and act as a stimulus for improved psychological care and for further research into this important and rapidly growing patient group.

Review of the literature

The literature on five main areas is reviewed. The scene is set with an overview of the 'state of the art' in liver transplantation. Four aspects of recovery from adult liver transplantation are then discussed:

(1) Psychiatric problems.
(2) Functional recovery.

(3) The psychological impact of 'unsuccessful' liver transplants.

(4) Quality of life.

A literature search was conducted which used a variety of sources: three computer databases were searched, the Cumulative Index of Nursing and Allied Health Literature and the Cumulative Index Medicus and psychological literature for the period 1983 to December 1994. Recent editions of journals were also searched.

Liver transplantation

The first human liver transplant was performed by Starzl at the University of Colorado, USA, in 1963 (Starzl *et al.* (1963). This first patient survived for 23 days, and it was a further five years before a patient survived for more than one year (Starzl *et al.* 1968). The first human liver transplant in the UK was performed in Cambridge in 1968 (Calne & Williams 1968). The one-year survival rate reached 30% in the late 1970s (Starzl *et al.* 1979). However, with the introduction of Cyclosporin, in 1980 a greater than 50% success rate was achieved (Starzl *et al.* 1981). In the USA the procedure was considered to be experimental until June 1983 when the National Institute of Health (NIH) declared that 'liver transplantation is a therapeutic modality for end-stage liver disease that deserves broader application' (National Institute of Health 1984).

After this slow start, liver transplantation has developed rapidly over the last decade. 'From 1963 to 1982, 466 liver transplants had been performed worldwide. In 1990 alone approximately 3000 liver transplants were performed worldwide, half of them in the United States' (Wright 1992). Liver transplantation has revolutionized hepatology as 'most patients with liver disease should be considered potential candidates for transplantation' (O'Grady & Williams 1988).

Survival rates have continued to improve. One year survival rates of 70–80% or higher are widely attained, with five-year survival rates of 60–70% (Bismuth *et al.* 1987). Currently, 'elective liver transplantation in low risk patients has a 90% one year survival' (Sherlock & Dooley 1993). The chances of a transplant-related death show a dramatic decline to 3% after the first year, so one-year survival represents a significant hurdle for patients (Iwatsuki *et al.* 1987). However, the goal of liver transplantation is not merely to prolong life but also to improve the patient's quality of life (Burroughs & Rolles 1990).

Liver transplantation 'is a tremendous undertaking that does not begin or end with the surgery' (Sherlock & Dooley 1993). Liver transplantation is 'the most time-consuming and costliest of all transplantations' (Hockerstedt 1990). Although the number of patients receiving liver transplantation in the

United Kingdom (UK) is small the British government is spending millions of pounds a year in this area. Promoting patient recovery and increasing their quality of life (QOL) is therefore an important area for future research.

The studies of recovery from liver transplantation have tended to look at four areas:

(1) Psychiatric aspects.
(2) Functional recovery.
(3) The psychological impact of 'unsuccessful' liver transplants.
(4) Quality of life.

Psychiatric aspects

Transplant candidates are carefully screened and selected and psychiatric assessment is generally an important part of this screening process. There are marked differences in practice between centres (Levenson & Olbrisch 1993). For example, in the UK alcohol dependence is generally regarded as a contraindication to liver transplantation (Neuberger 1989). In contrast, alcoholic patients are not excluded from transplant programmes in the USA. Survival rates are similar to non-alcoholics (Starzl *et el.* 1988), with only about one in 10 returning to alcohol misuse after transplantation (Kumar *et al.* 1989). Psychological and physical health are similar in alcoholic and non-alcoholic liver transplant recipients (Beresford *et al.* 1992; Knechtle *et al.* 1993).

Measures of the medical criteria for liver transplantation are well established (McCaughan, 1993). In contrast, assessment of psychosocial criteria is vague (Sigardson-Poor & Haggerty 1990). The development of the transplant evaluation rating scale (TERS), which classifies patients' levels of adjustment in ten areas of psychosocial functioning, is therefore a potentially important breakthrough. Retrospective ratings of 35 liver transplant patients showed that 'the TERS represents a promising instrument for transplant candidate selection as well as a valuable tool for further research' (Twillman *et al.* 1993).

Neuropsychological test deficits are expected in chronic liver disease (Sherlock & Dooley 1993). These impairments do improve but do not disappear after transplantation (Tarter *et al.* 1984; Tarter *et al.* 1990a). It has been shown that some patients have not returned to normal on such tests when assessed three years after liver transplantation (Tarter *et al.* 1988), and this can lower their QOL (Riether et al., 1992; Tarter et al., 1992). Short-term neuropsychiatric complications in hospitalised patients recovering from liver transplantation have been linked with drug toxicity (DiMartini *et al.*, 1991) and abnormal electrolyte levels (Della Monica *et al.*, 1993).

Trzepacz *et al.* (1986, 1989) and Trzepacz & DiMartini (1992) evaluated

247 liver transplant candidates in the USA and found half of them had a diagnostic and statistical manual-III diagnosis. They found 20% had an adjustment disorder, 19% delirium, 9% alcohol misuse, and 5% major depression. High levels of psychiatric morbidity led Surman *et al.* (1987) to argue that 'psychiatric consultation is an essential support to the transplant programme', as 24% of patients in their study of 40 post-transplant patients in Boston, USA, required treatment for depression and 7% for medical non-compliance. Similar levels of depression (one-third of 29 patients) have been found in a study of liver transplant patients in Holland (Heyink *et al.* 1990).

In the first study of the potential psychiatric needs of liver transplant patients in the UK (Commander *et al.* 1992), of the 32 patients in the study, 18.8% were found to have a psychiatric disorder on the psychiatric disorder on the psychiatric assessment schedule/research diagnostic criteria (PAS/RDC). This is comparable to that found in the general population in studies using this measure. Commander *et al.* (1992) conclude:

> 'the fact that only 50% of RDC cases were receiving treatment for their psychiatric disorder suggests that there is room for improvement in the psychiatric assessment and treatment of patients following this procedure.'

Research to evaluate the impact of psychiatric interventions on patient recovery from liver transplantation is needed (Collis & Lloyd 1992; Soos 1992; Surman 1992, 1994).

Functional recovery

Functional abilities include characteristics such as mobility, endurance, activities of daily living and employment. Esquivel *et al.* (1988) studied survival and functional recovery in 52 patients in the Pittsburgh series with primary biliary cirrhosis. They found that although 33% of respondents were working full-time after their liver transplant, 94% were able to care for themselves at home.

Robinson *et al.* (1990) surveyed patients three years after transplant in Pittsburgh, USA, and reported 39% of respondents in full-time employment, while a further 26% described themselves as homemakers. Only 48% could walk outside the house prior to transplant, but 94% could walk 'three blocks' after transplantation. Both mobility and endurance increased dramatically after transplantation. They conclude 'liver transplantation is returning a significant number of patients to an active, successful and satisfactory existence' (Robinson *et al.* 1990). However, these figures may not be an accurate representation of functional outcome after liver transplantation as only 45 of 95 patients were contacted and only 68% returned the postal questionnaire.

The results from the Mayo Clinic series in the USA are even more impressive, with Eid *et al.* (1989) reporting a 98% one-year survival rate. Of these 46 patients, 56% were employed and 35% were homemakers. Subjective wellbeing and satisfaction with life were reported by 91% of patients, according to a retrospective review of the patients' notes.

Lundgren *et al.* (1994) have examined the social ability and needs for medical care in a retrospective survey of 133 liver transplant patients in Huddinge, Sweden. Immediately before transplantation 73 patients (55%) were at home (of whom 22 were working) and 60 patients (45%) were in hospital. One year after transplant 95 patients (71%) were alive and of these survivors 87 patients (92%) were at home (of whom 61 were working), and eight patients were in hospital. Liver transplantation clearly diminishes the need for hospital medical care and enhances the capacity to work. A recent questionnaire survey of 346 liver transplant patients in the USA (with only a 48% response rate, *n* = 166) found all the patients could perform the activities of daily living (Nicholas *et al.* 1994).

The studies of functional recovery from liver transplantation indicate that the majority of patients who survive return to a more active lifestyle after the operation. However, the studies all adopt a rather simplistic approach. Future studies would benefit from a more complex research design. For example, functional abilities could be assessed using a standard tool, e.g. the Katz index of ADL (Katz *et al.* 1963), in a prospective longitudinal study.

Psychological impact of 'unsuccessful' liver transplantation

Researchers in Holland have examined the psychological needs of two categories of 'unsuccessful' liver transplant patients (Heyink *et al.* 1989; Tymstra 1989; Heyink & Tymstra 1990). In Groningen, 70% of candidates for liver transplantation are ultimately turned down, and 20–30% of adult patients die within the first year of their transplant. Expectations and hopes turn out to be illusions: the 'shadow side' of transplantation (Heyink & Tymstra 1990).

Liver transplantation not only has consequences for the successful transplant recipients but also for many others. Heyink & Tymstra (1990) interviewed the relatives of 16 patients who had died following liver transplantation. The mean patient survival was six months and relatives were interviewed, on average, a further three to eight years after this. One-third of the respondents felt that the patient would have been better off if they had not entered the programme. Moreover, over half found the loss more difficult to accept because the patient had been involved in the programme. Often 'the transplant is the last straw available for the liver patients to clutch at' (Tymstra 1989). As one of the patients Tymstra (1989) interviewed states, 'the choice between a chance of staying alive and certain death isn't really a choice'.

These research studies provide a poignant counterweight to the studies of the quality of life of the 'successful' liver transplant patients. It would seem worthwhile to combine both approaches in a large prospective study of recovery from liver transplantation.

Quality of life

Qualify of life has been described as a 'nebulous but essential outcome criterion' (Wilson-Barnett 1981). The concept has therefore proved difficult to define and measure (Goodinson & Singleton 1989). Quality of life is almost invariably mentioned in the title of papers which assess recovery from liver transplantation. The discussion of the literature which follows is therefore based on how various authors have labelled their own work.

At present there is only one published British study of quality of life (QOL) and liver transplantation (Lowe *et al*. 1990). In a review of QOL after organ transplantation Molzahn (1991) quotes four papers on liver transplantation (Tymstra *et al*. 1986; Esquivel *et al*. 1988; Tartar *et al*. 1988; Robinson *et al*. 1990). However, Molzahn's paper has two major shortcomings. First, it includes many studies that do not use a recognized generic or specific QOL measurement tool (e.g. Tymstra *et al*. 1986; Esquivel *et al*. 1988; Robinson *et al*. 1990). Second, the review of QOL and liver transplantation omits several important papers (Colonna *et al*. 1988; Lowe *et al*. 1990, Kober *et al*. 1990).

The initial reports of QOL and liver transplantation were retrospective (Colonna *et al*. 1988; Wolcott *et al*. 1989; Lowe *et al*. 1990; Felser *et al*. 1991). These represent the beginnings of a more detailed set of prospective studies of outcome that are necessary for the comprehensive evaluation of such programmes (McEwan 1991). A number of such prospective studies have now been published (Tarter *et al*. 1988; Kober *et al*. 1990; Kuchler *et al*. 1991; Tarter *et al*. 1991a; Bonsel *et al*. 1992; Moore *et al*. 1992a,b; Hicks *et al*. 1992).

Benefits of transplantation

Colonna *et al*. (1988) conducted a retrospective survey of 28 adult patients who had undergone liver transplantation at the University of California, Los Angeles (UCLA), USA. The results of the questionnaire they devised showed a dramatic increase in the patients QOL following liver transplantation. Forty-seven per cent found their QOL intolerable and 27% felt it was poor before the operation. In contrast, 67% rated their QOL as excellent after transplantation, 27% as good, 7% as satisfactory, and no one felt their QOL was either poor or intolerable.

In their cross-sectional retrospective survey of 81 patients in the Cambridge/Kings programme in March 1987, Lowe *et al*. (1990) found that on the Nottingham [England] Health Profile (NHP) their patients showed a QOL broadly similar to that of those of the same sex and age among the general population. The NHP was chosen as it had previously been used in the UK to demonstrate that the benefits of heart transplantation outweighed the costs (Buxton *et al.* 1985). Forty-seven per cent of the liver patients reported no problems with the six areas profiled in part I of the NHP. When these scores are compared with levels expected for community based age/sex norms, they represent a two-fold increase in problems with physical mobility but a 50% reduction in problems of emotional reaction in the transplant group. All other scores approximate the expected levels.

Responses to part II of the NHP showed a level of problems encountered similar to that expected in the general population. Lowe *et al.* (1990) suggest that post-transplant euphoria, a desire to demonstrate gratitude, or an over-reaction to their regained health may have had a positive effect on the patient's reported levels of health status.

> 'Many of the patients spontaneously wrote that the health profile questionnaire gave no opportunity to comment on the very positive feelings of wellbeing that they were experiencing … [which] reflects the dramatic improvements in perceived health of the liver transplant patients' (Lowe *et al.* 1990).

A research study which allows patients to talk about their experiences would therefore seem useful.

Kober *et al.* (1990) have recently reported an unusual two centre study. QOL is measured using the EORTC questionnaire. First, a cross-sectional study in Chicago compared the QOL of 38 liver transplant patients with 12 outpatients with chronic liver disease and 15 healthy individuals. The QOL of the liver transplant patients was significantly higher than for patients with chronic liver disease, and as high as healthy controls.

Second, a longitudinal study in Hamburg measured QOL 2, 6, 12, 24 and 36 months after transplant, with the following results:

(1) QOL only partly correlated with physical symptoms.
(2) There was a high correlation between rejection crisis periods and decreases on all QOL measures.
(3) In both samples men had a lower QOL than women. This seems to be influenced by three factors: men in the study exhibited more physical symptoms, poorer occupational rehabilitation and greater depression.
(4) Preoperative depression and lack of social support might be possible risk factors for long-term survival. In contrast, Tarter *et al.* (1990b) found no gender difference on measures of general health and psychosocial adjustment in 41 liver transplant patients. However, when they compared female spouses with male spouses, Tarter *et al.* (1990b) found

significantly greater stress and psychopathology amongst female spouses. These conflicting findings require further research.

(5) A psychotherapeutic support programme increases patient compliance and leads to better patient rehabilitation.

(6) All successfully transplanted patients show a significant postoperative increase in their overall QOL.

This study is important as it looks at changes in QOL over time. Previous studies have provided a one-off snapshot of QOL (Colonna *et al.* 1988; Wolcott *et al.* 1989; Lowe *et al.* 1990).

Another research group has presented these same results in a paper by Kuchler *et al.* (1991). Essentially, this is simply a shortened presentation of Kober *et al.* (1990). A longitudinal study in Hamburg, Germany, seems to be the only published study where an intervention designed to enhance patient recovery from liver transplantation has been tried. Unfortunately, Kober *et al.* (1990) and Kuchler *et al.* (1991) fail to specify what 'psychosocial support' their patients received. The absence of a control group of liver transplant patients is a further flaw in what purports to be an intervention study. A rigorously designed quasi-experimental study is therefore a potential area of future research.

Psychological measurement

Bonsel *et al.* (1992) have also combined cross-sectional ($n = 26$) and longitudinal ($n = 20$) data in an evaluation of QOL before and after liver transplantation in Holland. A wide range of psychological measurement scales were used including the state-trait anxiety inventory, the self rating depression scale, the Karnofsky index, and the Nottingham health profile. Bonsel *et al.* (1992) give an impressive table of mean scores for these scales for the general population and liver patients pre-transplant and post-transplant (at four separate times). Unfortunately, the value of the discussion of their table is severely limited as it is not based on a statistical analysis of these data. The authors conclude: 'a comparison with the NHP scores as reported by Lowe *et al.* (1990) shows close similarity of the post-transplant results' (Bonsel *et al.* 1992).

QOL is often seen as an evaluation of the individual's subjective life satisfaction in contract to the more 'objective' measures of functional capacity (Tarter *et al.* 1988). In Pittsburgh, USA, patients undergo a battery of psychological tests (taking approximately four hours) prior to placement on the liver transplantation waiting list. Cognitive ability, emotional stability and social adjustment are all measured.

In a two-year prospective study of 66 liver transplantation patients. Tarter *et al.* (1988) examined QOL (sickness impact profile, SIP), coping (ways of coping scale), stress (hassles scale), psychological adjustment (symptom checklist), and social support (social behaviour assessment schedule, SBAS). It was found that 43% had no problem performing their job. Forty-eight per cent rated their QOL as 'good', 37% 'excellent' and only 1% rated it as 'poor'. Of the 66 subjects, 9% had a negative appraisal of self-worth; 12% felt angry and 11% felt depressed. On the subscales of the SIP the greatest improvements relative to their pre-transplant scores were observed on scales measuring alertness (27% improvement), general psychosocial functioning (17%), and home management (25%). Sixty-five per cent of the patients were concerned about their health and continued to monitor it closely.

The extent to which the patient's and spouse's adjustments are related post-transplant was also studied. Unfortunately the presentation of this by Tarter *et al.* (1988) is unclear. No sample size is given (?$n=66$), no tables are produced, and there is no discussion of these findings: just a series of correlations in the results section. Some of the same battery of psychological tests seem to be given to both patient and spouse post-transplant, i.e. ways of coping, hassles scale, and the symptom checklist. The researchers found that the stress experienced by the spouse correlated with some of the patient's characteristics. For example, the greater the number of emotional symptoms reported by the patient the greater the stress experienced by the spouse. Other variables which correlated with 'spousal stress' include patient anxiety, patient stress, daily hassles experienced by the patient, and perceived level of family support.

Few of these correlations reach conventional levels of statistical significance, but they do suggest that the wellbeing of patient and spouse are entwined.

'It remains to be determined whether the prognosis in patients with high stress, low social support, and spousal stress differs from that of transplant patients who have a less stressful environment' (Tarter *et al.* 1988).

Tarter *et al.* (1988) conclude:

'Liver transplantation surgery results in a sharp improvement in quality of life relative to one's pretransplant status, although it does not return the recipient to their premorbid baseline.'

Impact of liver disease

Tarter *et al.* (1991b) have administered the SIP to 306 prospective adult liver transplant patients in Pittsburgh. This large sample enabled them to examine the differential impact of eight chronic liver diseases on QOL. This is the first study to investigate whether or not disease specific impairments exist. 'It is interesting to note that for every disease type, the psychosocial impact of their disease was perceived as being more severe than the physical consequences of their disease' (Tarter *et al.* 1991b). This has implications when developing patient teaching/rehabilitation programmes.

Moreover, the physical and psychosocial impact of disease was not associated with the severity of the liver disease (i.e. insignificant chi-squared analysis of SIP versus Child's index of liver disease). They also found no significant difference in QOL between those with alcoholic cirrhosis and other liver diseases. This research suggests that combining patients with different types and severities of chronic liver diseases when examining the psychosocial impact of liver transplantation is a valid research strategy.

Tarter *et al.* (1991a) have recently improved on the design of their 1988 study. Fifty-three non-alcoholic patients with advanced chronic liver disease were evaluated prior to and three years after liver transplantation using the SIP and the SBAS. A group of 35 'normal control individuals' were also evaluated to establish a baseline level of normal functioning at a similar test–retest interval. The SBAS was also administered to 'informants' (i.e. the spouses or parents) of both groups of 'subjects'. The SBAS 'not only documents the patient's quality of social adjustment but also that of family members with the explicit objective of linking any identified social adjustment disturbances to the disease status of the patient' (Tarter *et al.* 1991a).

Comparisons between the two informant groups prior to transplant revealed significant disturbances in the transplantation subjects on the subscales of the SBAS measuring disturbed behaviour, social performance and burden on the family. Despite these statistically significant levels of psychosocial disruption in both transplant subjects and their significant others, 'distress in the informant caused by the burden placed on the family did not discriminate the transplant recipients from the control group' (Tarter *et al.* 1991a). On re-evaluation after transplantation there was no statistical difference between the control group and liver group on any of the SBAS scales. Significant improvements were found for the liver group which eroded all of their pre-transplant deficits.

At the time of pre-transplant assessment the liver transplant group were significantly impaired ($P < 0.001$) on all of the 12 SIP scales compared with the control group. The liver transplant recipients were significantly impaired on eight of the SIP scales post-transplant (ambulation, social interaction, communication, alertness, sleep and rest, eating, work and recreation). However, a large and significant improvement from pre-transplant to post-transplant was found on all scales except work capacity. A 70.2% improvement was found on the scales measuring the psychosocial dimension of the SIP, and a 89.5% improvement on the physical dimension.

Improvement in health status

Tarter *et al.* (1991a) found both the patient and their informant reported on almost universal improvement in health status following liver transplantation. The differences in the results from the SIP and SBAS may be due to several factors. The SIP may be a more sensitive instrument and therefore detect more impairment than the SBAS and the self-report format of the SIP may give a more accurate picture of the patient's condition than the informant report of the SBAS. The mean severity of impairment across all 12 scales of the SIP was only 5.2%. 'Despite being impaired statistically compared with normal control subjects, the absolute magnitude of the residual disturbance is modest, indicating that the impairment may not be important clinically' (Tarter *et al.* 1991a).

The researchers warn of the dangers of only considering group scores which often obscure large individual differences, and recommend further research on this subset of 'problem' patients. This will enable rehabilitation to be targeted at those with persisting impairments, and also help to identify potential recipients who are likely to experience the maximal improvement in their QOL following liver transplantation. Similar aims have guided research on recovery following major cardiac surgery (West & Wilson-Barnett 1989).

Moore *et al.* (1992a, 1992b) have published two brief reports of the beginnings of a comprehensive evaluation of QOL following liver transplantation at the Austin Hospital, Australia. Moore *et al.* (1992a) present a short discussion of results on nine liver transplant patients and nine control patients (the nature of the control group is not given). 'A battery of standardized psychological assessments is administered which includes Profile of Mood States (POMS), Quality of Life Scale (LASA), Wechsler Adult Intelligence Test (WAIS-R), Wechsler Memory Scale (WMS), Complex Figure of Rey, Benton, Controlled Oral Word Test, and a series of personality scales' (Moore *et al.* 1992a). Data were gathered preoperatively and at one, three and nine months postoperatively for both groups. The authors report improvements in mood state, cognitive functioning and QOL as early as one month post-transplant, with further improvements at three and nine months post-transplant.

No improvements were found in the control group. Unfortunately, the statistical significance of these results is omitted.

Moore *et al.* (1992b) do report the statistical significance of their results in their later paper. However, it is unclear if the 22 liver transplant patients and 11 controls (non-alcoholic cirrhotic patients) in this second report includes any of the patients from their earlier paper (Moore *et al.* 1992a). Their second paper reports the results of two other psychological measurements: the psychological adjustment to illness scale (PAIS) and the Austin QOL scale (AUSQUAL). They state that AUSQUAL is unpublished, but provide no information on the reliability and validity of this scale. Data were collected at the same time intervals as in Moore *et al.* (1992a). Both control and transplant groups were statistically equivalent at baseline. There was no significant change in the scores of the control group. Liver transplant patients showed a significant improvement ($P < 0.001$) in their QOL even one month post-transplant.

Some of the shortcomings in the two papers by Moore *et al.* (1992a, 1992b) may be ascribed to their brevity (one page each). However, if complex research studies are to benefit other researchers then it is important that such studies are reported comprehensively. Brevity makes clarity imperative. Inadequate reporting of the rationale of complex studies may damage the reputation of quantitative research. This type of approach to research has been described by Morse (1992) as amounting to little more than a 'multivariate scaling "fishing trip" '.

Comparison with other health-related variables

A recent study has compared QOL and other health-related variables in two groups of liver transplant patients (Hicks *et al.* 1992). Two years is used as a watershed to divide the mid-western sample into 'short-term' ($n = 18$) and 'long-term' ($n = 17$) patients. Seventy-three per cent of the 48 patients who were invited to participate in the study returned a questionnaire which included the SIP, a visual analogue scale of perceived health status. The profile of mood states (POMS), and the quality of life index-liver transplant (QLI-LT). The QLI-LT was modified from the original QLI (Ferrans & Powers 1985) by adding two items, on satisfaction with the liver transplant and freedom from pain, to each of the four QLI subscales (health and function, socioeconomic, psychological/spiritual and family). Each of the four domains is weighted for importance to the individual and so the patient's perceived quality of life is measured (i.e. importance × satisfaction), not just their degree of satisfaction (Ferrans & Powers 1985).

The long-term group reported higher levels of functional impairment on the physical dimension of the SIP and on the total SIP. The two groups had similar scores on perceived health status, with means above average. There were no significant differences between the groups on POMS, nor on any of its subscales. No significant differences were found between groups on the QLI-LT scale. The mean overall QOL of this sample was similar to the mean reported for a healthy control group measured with the QLI (Ferrans & Powers 1985). 'Almost all patients stated that the reason the transplant had been worth it was because it bought them more time with their families' (Hicks *et al.* 1992). The authors suggest that future studies should 'describe other factors', but fail to mention what these could be.

The studies of QOL after liver transplantation show a degree of methodological sophistication that is lacking in the studies of both psychiatric problems and functional recovery in this patient group. A critique of these complex research studies is presented in the discussion section below.

Discussion

The literature on psychological recovery from liver transplantation continues to grow. Early studies on patient's functional recovery (Esquivel *et al.* 1988; Eid *et al.* 1989; Robinson *et al.* 1990; Lundgren *et al.* 1994; Nicholas *et al.* 1994) have been superseded by a series of studies which seek to assess the patient's quality of life (QOL). These QOL research studies have also moved on from a retrospective approach in the earlier studies (Colonna *et al.* 1988; Wolcott *et al.* 1989; Lowe *et al.* 1990; Felser *et al.* 1991; Leyendecker *et al.* 1993; Chen & Sun 1994) to prospective designs in most recent literature (Tarter *et al.* 1988; Kober *et al.* 1990; Kuchler *et al.* 1991; Tarter *et al.* 1991a; Tarter *et al.* 1991b; Bonsel *et al.* 1992; Moore *et al.* 1992a; Hicks *et al.* 1992).

Leyendecker *et al.* (1993) assessed psychological status, social support and QOL using a range of instruments, in a cross-sectional pilot study of 45 liver transplant patients in Berlin, Germany. Average follow-up time was nine months post-transplant. Sixty per cent of patients reported their QOL to be very high, 31% medium and 9% felt very bad. Patients with extra-hepatic diseases had the lowest QOL.

Chen & Sun (1994) used patient self assessment to evaluate the QOL of seven liver transplant patients in Taiwan. They conclude: 'not only is liver transplantation a life-saving procedure for patients with end-stage liver disease, it is also a means by which 'health' can be achieved in the way defined by the WHO in 1947'.

The research design has also tended to become increasingly complex. Single 'instrument' studies on a single group (Esquivel *et al.* 1988; Eid *et al.* 1989; Robinson *et al.* 1990; Lowe *et al.* 1990) have been followed by multiple instrument studies on several groups (Tarter *et al.* 1988; Kober *et al.* 1990; Kuchler *et al.* 1991; Tarter *et al.* 1991a; Bonsel *et al.* 1992; Moore *et al.* 1992a,b; Hicks *et al.* 1992). Unfortunately, only one UK study has been published and this uses a retrospective single instrument approach. In contrast, Tarter's multidisciplinary research team in Pittsburgh, USA, has done far more than any other group to increase our knowledge of psychosocial adjustment following liver transplantation. Hopefully, researchers in the UK will eventually develop a comprehensive research programme to investigate the psychosocial needs of this important patient group.

Generic instruments

The research on QOL and liver transplantation is dominated by the use of generic rather than disease specific instruments. Both the NHP and SIP have the advantage of being well tested (McDowell & Newell 1987; Fallowfield 1990; Bowling 1991; Gill & Feinstein 1994; Bowling 1995). In addition, their extensive use allows comparison between liver transplant studies and also with studies of other disease groups. Although the breadth of generic instruments allows for the detection of unexpected effects, such a broad approach may reduce responsiveness to the effects of health care. The advantages and disadvantages of disease specific instruments are the opposite to those of the generic instruments (Fletcher *et al.* 1992).

Disease specific tools potentially reduce the burden placed on patients and increase patient acceptability by including only relevant dimensions. Disadvantages are lack of comparability of results with those from other disease groups, and the possibility of missing effects in dimensions that are not included. For the researcher examining QOL and liver transplantation there is only one published specific instrument available (Hicks *et al.* 1992). Perhaps even this is not very specific as it was developed from a tool to measure QOL in haemodialysis patients (Ferrans & Powers 1985) by adding two questions related to liver transplantation. Research to develop a comprehensive tool to measure QOL in liver transplant patients is required.

The concept of quality of life

One of the major problems with QOL is that nearly every researcher has defined the concept differently (Diener 1984; Goodinson & Singleton 1989; Meeberg 1993). Although 'the definition of the concept remains elusive' (Dean 1992), QOL has been equated with life satisfaction, self-esteem, wellbeing, health, happiness, adjustment, functional status, value of life and even the meaning of life (Dean 1992). Attempts to refine the concept have often resulted in one nebulous concept being replaced by several different but equally nebulous concepts. For example, Zhan (1992) proposed a 'conceptual model' of QOL. She suggests that four aspects are essential for an assessment of QOL: life satisfaction, self-concept, health, and social wellbeing. Such an approach has been countermanded by nurses who adopt a phenomenological perspective (Benner 1985) and see attempts to measure QOL as 'expressive of a fractured and reductionist view of what it means to be a human being' (Draper 1992).

Conclusion

Although there is a great deal of quantitative research on recovery from acute illness and on living with chronic illness, much of this fails to capture the patient's own experience of illness (Morse & Johnson 1991). 'To a patient an illness is an experience, not easily reduced to a list of variables measured in the laboratory or clinic' (Sensky & Catalan 1992). Numerous 'psychosocial' measures have been used to describe the QOL of liver transplant patients. However, the process of adjustment and the personal experiences of liver transplant patients are not very well understood. A qualitative approach may prove to be more illuminating, and can act as an indirect assessment of a patient's overall 'quality of life'. Such an approach circumnavigates, rather than surmounts the considerable problems of defining and measuring QOL.

Wainwright (1993, 1995) used in-depth focused interviews with ten patients to describe the experiences of liver transplantation from the patient's perspective. The living hell of life before their transplant was replaced at around one year after transplant by an almost euphoric sense of wellness; their lives were transformed. Informants felt the medical and nursing care they received from the hospital was excellent. However, the patients seemed to discover more information about the experience of liver transplantation from other patients than from health professionals. Nurses therefore need to take a more active role in teaching patients. In addition, the support patients give each other should be encouraged, for example by developing patient support groups (Doherty 1994).

There is a need for more research into the nurses' role in enhancing the quality of life of both liver transplant patients and their families. Recent reviews have called for more evaluation research into the efficacy of the psychological interventions of specialist nurses in general (Wilson-Barnett & Beech 1994; Wilson-Barnett 1995) and of liver transplant clinical nurse specialists in particular (Benning & Smith, 1994).

Although the quantitative studies of recovery from liver transplantation have become more ambitious, none attempt to place patient recovery in a theoretical framework. Many previous studies of recovery from illness (e.g. Webb 1983) have used the conceptual framework of stress and coping developed by Lazarus (Lazarus 1966; Lazarus & Folkman 1984). Using the Lazarus model as a framework for research on this group of patients seems worthwhile. As the Lazarus model uses a person-centred approach, Morse & Johnson (1991) argue that this is congruent with their 'illness-constellation model', which is a synthesis of five grounded theory studies of the experience of illness.

'It seems possible that triangulation will be the research trend of the 90s' (Burns & Grove 1993). A large scale research study which attempts to integrate quantitative and qualitative data on recovery from liver transplantation would therefore seem appropriate. Moreover, the combined use of the Lazarus (1966) model as the framework for the quantitative parts of such a study and the Morse & Johnson (1991) model as a framework for the qualitative aspects of the study, could lead to theoretical developments that have implications for studies of patient recovery and of patient experiences of illness in general.

References

Benner, P. (1985) Quality of life: a phenomenological perspective on explanation, prediction and understanding in nursing science. *Advances in Nursing Science*, **8**(1), 1–14.

Benning, C.R. & Smith, A. (1994) Psychosocial needs of family members of liver transplant patients. *Clinical Nurse Specialist*, **8**, 280–88.

Beresford, T.P., Scwartz, J., Wilson, D., Merion, R. & Lucey, M.R. (1992) The short-term psychological health of alcoholic and non-alcoholic liver transplant recipients. *Alcoholism, Clinical & Experimental Research*, **16**, 996–1000.

Bismuth, H., Castaing, D., Otte, J.B., Rolles, K., Ringe, B. & Slooff, M. (1987) Hepatic transplantation in Europe. *Lancet*, **II**, 674–6.

Bonsel, G.J., Essink-Bot, M.L., Klompmaker, I.J. & Slooff, M.J.H. (1992) Assessment of the quality of life before and following liver transplantation. *Transplantation*, **53**, 796–800.

Bowling, A. (1991) *Measuring Health: a Review of Quality of Life Measurement Scales*. Oxford University Press, Milton Keynes.

Bowling, A. (1995) *Measuring Disease: a review of specific quality of life measurement scales*. Open University Press, Milton Keynes.

Burns, N. & Grove, S.K. (1993) *The Practice of Nursing Research: Conduct, Critique and Utilization*, 2nd edn. Saunders, Philadelphia.

Burroughs, A.K. & Rolles, K. (1990) Liver transplantation. In *Recent Advances in Gastroenterology* (Ed R. Pounder), vol. 8, pp. 179–98. Churchill Livingstone, London.

Buxton, M., Acheson, R.M., Caine, N., Gibson, S. & O'Brian, B. (1985) *Costs and Benefits of the Heart Transplant Programme at Harefield and Papworth Hospitals*. HMSO London.

Calne, R.Y. & Williams, R. (1968) Liver transplantation in man-I. Observations on technique and organisation in five cases. *British Medical Journal*, **280**, 535–40.

Chen, C.L. & Sun, C.K. (1994) Quality of life following orthoptic liver transplantation. *Transplantation Proceedings*, **26**, 2266–8.

Collis, I. & Lloyd, G. (1992) Psychiatric aspects of liver disease. *British Journal of Psychiatry*, **161**, 12–22.

Colonna, J.O., Brems, J.J., Hiatt, J.R., Millis, J.M., Ament, M.E., Baldrich-Quinones, W.J., Berequist, W.E., Besbris, D., Brill, J.E., Goldstein, L.I., Nuesse, B.J., Ramming, K.P., Saleh, S., Vargas, J.H. & Busuttil, R.W. (1988) The quality of survival after liver transplantation. *Transplantation Proceedings*, XX, 594–7.

Commander, M., Neuberger, J. & Dean, C. (1992) Psychiatric and social consequences of liver transplantation. *Transplantation*, **53**, 1038–40.

Dean, H. (1992) Multiple instruments for measuring quality of life. In *Instruments for clinical nursing research* (Ed. M. Frank-Stromberg), 97–106. Jones & Bartlett, Boston.

Della Monica, O., Alfani, D., Berloco, P., Bruzzone, P., Caricato, M., Marciani, A., Rossi, M. Urbano, D. & Cortesini, R. (1993) Neuropsychiatric complications after liver transplantation: a single centre experience. *Transplantation Proceedings*, **25**, 1771–2.

Diener, E. (1984) Subjective well-being. *Psychological Bulletin*, **95**, 542–75.

DiMartini, A., Pajer, K., Trzepacz, P., Fung, J., Starzl, T. & Tringali, R. (1991) Psychiatric morbidity in liver transplant patients. *Transplantation Proceedings*, **23**, 3179–80.

Doherty, P. (1994) Patient and family support groups: what is their role? In *Quality of Life Following Renal Failure: Psychosocial Challenges accompanying High Technology Medicine* (Eds H.M. McGee & C. Bradley), pp. 259–64. Harwood Academic Publishers, Lausanne.

Draper, P. (1992) Quality of life as quality of being: an alternative to the subject–object dichotomy. *Journal of Advanced Nursing*, **17**, 965–70.

Eid, A., Steffen, R., Porayko, M.K., Beers, T.R., Kaese, D.E., Wiesner, R.H. & Krom, R.A.F. (1989) Beyond one year after liver transplantation. *Mayo Clinic Proceedings*, **64**, 446–50.

Esquivel, C.O., Van Thiel, D.H. Demetris, A.J., Berbardos, A., Iwatsuki, S., Markus, B., Gordon, R.D., Wallis North, J., Makowka, L., Tzakis, A.G., Todo, S., Gavaaler, J.S. & Starzl, T.E. (1988) Transplantation for primary biliary cirrhosis. *Gastroenterology*, **94**, 1207–16.

Fallowfield, L. (1990) *The Quality of Life*. Souvenir, London.

Felser, I., Wagner, S., Depee, J., Johnson, N., Staschak, S., Jain, A., Fung, J.J. & Starzl, T.E. (1991) Changes in the quality of life following conversion from CyA to FK 506 in orthotopic liver transplant patients. *Transplantation Proceedings*, **23**, 3032–4.

Ferrans, C.E. & Powers, M. (1985) Quality of life index: development and psychometric properties. *Advances in Nursing Science*, **8**, 15–24.

Fletcher, A., Gore, S., Jones, D., Fitzpatrick, R., Spiegelhalter, D. & Cox, D. (1992) Quality of life measures in health care, II: design, analysis, and interpretation. *British Medical Journal*, **305**, 1145–8.

Gill, T.M. & Feinstein, A.R. (1994) A critical appraisal of the quality-of-life measurements. *Journal of the American Medical Association*, **272**, 619–26.

Goodinson, S.M. & Singleton, J. (1989) Quality of life: a critical review of current concepts, measures, and their clinical implications. *International Journal of Nursing Studies*, **26**, 327–41.

Heyink, J.W. & Tymstra, T. (1990) Liver transplantation: the shadow side. *Family Practice*, **7**, 233–7.

Heyink, J.W., Tymstra, T.J., Van den Heuvel, W.J.A., Slooff, M.J.H. & Klompmaker, I.J. (1989) Liver transplantation: the rejected patients. *Transplantation*, **6**, 1069–71.

Heyink, J.W., Tymstra, T., Slooff, M.J.H. & Klompmaker, I. (1990) Liver transplantation – psychosocial problems following the operation. *Transplantation*, **49**, 1018–19.

Hicks, F.D., Larson, J.L. & Ferrans, C.E. (1992) Quality of life after liver transplant. *Research in Nursing & Health*, **15**, 111–19.

Hokerstedt, K. (1990) Liver Transplantation Today. *Scandinavian Journal of Gastroenterology*, **25**, 1–10.

Iwatsuki, S., Starzl, T.E., Gordon, R.D., Esquivel, C.O., Todo, S., Tzakis, A.G., Makowka, L., Marsh, J.W. Jr. & Miller, C.M. (1987) Late mortality and morbidity after liver transplantation. *Transplantation Proceedings*, **19**, 2373–7.

Katz, S., Ford, A.B., Moskowitz, R.W., Jackson, B.A. & Jaffe, M.W. (1963) Studies of illness in the aged. *Journal of the American Medical Association*, **185**, 914–18.

Knechtle, S.J., Fleming, M.F., Barry, K.L., Steen, D., Pirsch, J.D., D'Alessandro, A.M., Kalayoglu, M. & Belzer, F.O. (1993) Liver transplantation in alcoholics: assessment of psychological health and work activity. *Transplantation Proceedings*, **25**, 1916–18.

Kober, B., Kuchler, T., Broelsch, C., Kremer, B. & Henne-Bruns, D. (1990) A psychological support concept and quality of life research in a liver transplantation program: an interdisciplinary multicentre study. *Psychotherapy and Psychosomatics*, **54**, 117–31.

Kuchler, T., Kober, B., Broelsch, C., Henne-Bruns, D. & Kremer, B. (1991) Quality of life after liver transplantation: can a psychosocial support program contribute? *Transplantation Proceedings*, **23**, 1541–4.

Kumar, S., Basista, M., Stauber, R.E., Gavaler, J.S., Dindzans, V.J., Schade, R.R., Rabinovitz, M., Tarter, R.E. & Van Thiel, D.H. (1989) Orthotopic liver transplantation for alcoholic liver disease. *Gastroenterology*, **96**, A616.

Lazarus, R.S. (1966) *Psychological Stress and the Coping Process*. McGraw-Hill, New York.

Lazarus, R.S. & Folkman, S. (1984) *Stress, Appraisal and Coping*. Springer, New York.

Levenson, J.L. & Olbrisch, M.E. (1993) Psychosocial evaluation of organ transplant candidates: a comparative survey of process, criteria, and outcomes in heart, liver, and kidney transplantation. *Psychosomatics*, **34**, 314–23.

Leyendecker, B., Bartholomew, U. Neuhaus, R., Horhold, M., Blumhardt, G. Neuhaus, P. & Klapp, B.F. (1993) Quality of life of liver transplant recipients: a pilot study. *Transplantation*, **56**, 561–7.

Lowe, D., O'Grady, J.G., McEwen, J. & Williams, R. (1990) Quality of life following liver transplantation: preliminary report. *Journal of The Royal College of Physicians of London*, **24**, 43–6.

Lundgren, M., Kristiansson, M., Ericzon, B.G. & Eleborg, L. (1994) Improved quality of life after liver transplantation. *Transplantation Proceedings*, **26**, 1779.

McCaughan, G.W. (1993) Selection of patients for liver transplantation. *Journal of Gastroenterology and Hepatology*, **8**, 185–94.

McDowell, I. & Newell, C. (1987) *Measuring Health: A Guide to Rating Scales and Questionnaires*. Oxford University Press, Oxford.

McEwen, J. (1991) Health profile of liver transplant survivors. *Hospital Update*, March, 171–2.

Meeberg, G.A. (1993) Quality of life: a concept analysis. *Journal of Advanced Nursing*, **18**, 32–8.

Molzahn, A.E. (1991) Quality of life after organ transplantation. *Journal of Advanced Nursing*, **16**, 1042–7.

Moore, K.A., Burrows, G., Jones, R. McL. & Hardy, K. (1992a) Control evaluation of cognitive functioning, mood state, and quality of life post-liver transplant. *Transplantation Proceedings*, **24**, 202.

Moore, K.A., Jones, R. McL, Angus, P., Hardy, K. & Burrows, G. (1992b) Psychosocial adjustment to illness: quality of life following liver transplantation. *Transplantation Proceedings*, **24**, 2257–8.

Morse, J.M. & Johnson, J.L. (Eds) (1991) *The Illness Experience: Dimensions of Suffering*. Sage, Newbury Park, California.

Morse, J.M. (Ed) (1992) *Qualitative Health Research*. Sage, Newbury Park, California.

National Institute of Health (1984) Consensus Development Conference Statement: Liver Transplantation. June 20–23, 1983. *Hepatology*, **4**(1) Supplement, 107S–110S.

Neuberger, J.M. (1989) Transplantation for alcoholic liver disease. *British Medical Journal*, **299**, 693–4.

Nicholas, J.J., Oleske, D., Robinson, L.R., Switala, J.A. & Tarter, R. (1994) The quality of life after orthotopic liver transplantation: an analysis of 166 cases. *Archives of Physical Medicine & Rehabilitation*, **75**, 431–5.

O'Grady, J. & Williams, R. (1988) Present position of liver transplantation and its impact on hepatological practice. *Gut*, **29**, 566–70.

Riether, A.M., Smith, S.L., Lewison, B.J., Cotsonis, G.A. & Epstein, C.M. (1992) Quality-of-life changes and psychiatric and neurocognitive outcome after heart and liver transplantation. *Transplantation*, **54**, 444–50.

Robinson, L.R., Switala, J., Tarter, R.E. & Nichols, J.J. (1990) Functional outcome after liver transplantation: a preliminary report. *Archives of Physical Medical Rehabilitation*, **71**, 426–7.

Sensky, T. & Catalan, J. (1992) Asking patients about their treatment. *British Medical Journal*, **305**, 1109–10.

Sherlock, S. & Dooley, J. (1993) *Diseases of the Liver and Biliary System*, 9th Edn. Blackwell Science, Oxford.

Sigardson-Poor, K.M. & Haggerty, L.M. (Eds) (1990) *Nursing care of the transplant recipient*. Saunders, Philadelphia.

Soos, J. (1992) Psychotherapy and counselling with transplant patients. In *Psychiatric aspects of organ transplantation* (Eds J. Craven & G.M. Rodin), pp. 89–107. Oxford University Press, Oxford.

Starzl, T.E., Marchioro, T.L., Von Kaulla, K.N., Hermann, G., Brittain, R.S. & Waddell, W.R. (1963) Homotransplantation of the liver in humans. *Surgery, Gynecology & Obstetrics*, **117**, 659–65.

Starzl, T.E., Groth, C.G., Brettschneider, L., Penn, I., Fulgitini, V.A., Moon, J.B., Blanchard, H., Martin, A.J. & Porter, K.A. (1968) Orthotopic homotransplantation of the human liver. *Annals of Surgery*, **168**, 392–8.

Starzl, T.E., Koep, L.J., Halgrimson, C.G. & Hood, J. (1979) Fifteen years of clinical liver transplantation. *Gastroenterology*, **77**, 375–80.

Starzl, T.E., Klintmalm, G.B., Porter, K.A. & Iwatsuki, S. (1981) Liver transplantation with use of cyclosporin A and prednisone. *New England Journal of Medicine*, **205**, 366–8.

Starzl, T.E., Van Thiel, D.H., Tzakis, A.G., Shunzaburo, I., Todo, S., Wallis Marsh, J., Staschak, S., Stieber, A. & Gordon, R.D. (1988) Orthotopic Liver Transplantation for Alcoholic Cirrhosis. *Journal of the American Medical Association*, **260**, 2542–4.

Surman, O.S. (1992) Liver Transplantation. In *Psychiatric aspects of organ transplantation* (Eds J. Craven & G.M. Rodin), pp. 177–88. Oxford University Press, Oxford.

Surman, O.S. (1994) Psychiatric aspects of liver transplantation. *Psychosomatics*, **35**, 297–307.

Surman, O.S., Dienstag, J.L., Cosimi, A.B., Chauncey, S. & Russell, P.S. (1987) Psychosomatic aspects of liver transplantation. *Psychotherapy and Psychosomatics*, **48**, 26–31.

Tarter, R.E., Van Thiel, D.H. Hegedus, A.M., Schade, R.R., Gavaler, J.S. & Starzl, T.E. (1984) Neuropsychiatric status after liver transplantation. *Journal of Laboratory and Clinical Medicine*, **103**, 776–82.

Tarter, R.E., Erb, S., Biller, P.A., Switiala, J. & Van Thiel, D.H. (1988) The quality of life following liver transplantation: a preliminary report. *Gastroenterology Clinics of North America*, **17**, 207–17.

Tarter, R.E., Switala, J., Arria, A., Plail, J. & Van Thiel, D.H. (1990a) Subclinical hepatic encephalopathy: comparison before and after orthotopic liver transplantation. *Transplantation*, **50**, 632–7.

Tarter, R.E., Switala, J., Kabene, M. & Van Thiel, D.H. (1990b) Long-term psychosocial adjustment following liver transplantation: gender comparisons of patients and their spouses. *Family Systems Medicine*, **8**, 359–64.

Tarter, R.E., Switala, J., Arria, A., Plail, J. & Van Thiel, D.H. (1991a) Quality of life before and after orthotopic hepatic transplantation. *Archives of Internal Medicine*, **151**, 1521–6.

Tarter, R.E., Switala, J., Arria, A. & Van Thiel, D.H. (1991b) Impact of liver disease on daily living in transplantation candidates. *Journal of Clinical Epidemiology*, **44**, 1079–83.

Tarter, R.E., Switala, J., Plail, J. Havrilla, J. & Van Thiel, D.H. (1992) Severity of hepatic encephalopathy before liver transplantation is associated with quality of life after transplantation. *Archives of Internal Medicine*, **152**, 2097–101.

Trzepacz, P.T., Maue, F.R. & Coffmam, G. (1986) Neuropsychiatric assessment of liver transplantation candidates: delirium and other psychiatric disorders. *International Journal of Psychiatry in Medicine*, **16**, 101–11.

Trzepacz, P.T., Brenner, R. & Van Thiel, D.H. (1989) A psychiatric study of 247 liver transplantation candidates. *Psychosomatics*, **30**, 147–53.

Trzepacz, P.T. & DiMartini, A. (1992) Survival of 247 liver transplant candidates: relationship to pretransplant psychiatric variables and presence of delirium. *General Hospital Psychiatry*, **14**, 380–86.

Twillman, R.K., Manetto, C., Wellisch, D.K. & Wolcott, D.L. (1993) The transplant evaluation rating scale: a revision of the psychosocial levels system for evaluating organ transplant candidates. *Psychosomatics*, **34**, 144–53.

Tymstra, T.J., Bucking, J. Roorda, J., Van den Heuvel, W.J.A. & Gips, C.H. (1986) The psychosocial impact of a liver transplant programme. *Liver*, **6**, 302–9.

Tymstra, T.J. (1989) The imperative character of medical technology and the meaning of 'anticipated decision regret'. *International Journal of Technology Assessment in Health Care*, **5**, 207–13.

Wainwright, S.P. (1993) Getting a second chance: a grounded theory study of the transformational experience of liver transplantation. Unpublished MSc Dissertation, King's College London, University of London.

Wainwright, S.P. (1995) The transformational experience of liver transplantation. *Journal of Advanced Nursing*, **22**, 6.

Webb, C. (1983) A study of recovery from hysterectomy. In *Nursing Research: 10 Studies in Patient Care* (Ed. J. Wilson-Barnett), pp. 195–228. Wiley, New York.

West, S. & Wilson-Barnett, J. (1989) Risk Factors and Recovery from Coronary Artery Bypass Surgery. In *Directions in Nursing Research: Ten Years of Progress at London University* (Eds J. Wilson-Barnett & S. Robinson), pp. 117–125. Scutari Press, London.

Wilson-Barnett, J. (1981) Assessment of recovery: with special reference to a study with postoperative cardiac patients. *Journal of Advanced Nursing*, **6**, 435–45.

Wilson-Barnett, J. (1995) Specialism in nursing: effectiveness and maximization of benefit. *Journal of Advanced Nursing*, **21**, 1–2.

Wilson-Barnett, J. & Beech, S. (1994) Evaluating the clinical nurse specialist: a literature review. *International Journal of Nursing Studies*, **31**, 561–71.

Wolcott, D., Norquist, G. & Busuttil, R. (1989) Cognitive function and quality of life in adult liver transplant recipients. *Transplantation Proceedings*, **21**, 3563.

Wright, T.L. (1992) Medical aspects of liver transplantation. In *Wright's Liver and Biliary Disease* (Eds G.H. Millward-Sadler, R. Wright & M.J.P. Arthur), 3rd edn, Vol. II, pp. 1147–60. Saunders, Philadelphia.

Zhan, L. (1992) Quality of life: conceptual and measurement issues. *Journal of Advanced Nursing*, **17**, 795–800.

Chapter 10
Intensive care: situations of ethical difficulty

ANNA SÖDERBERG, *RNT*
Doctoral Student, Department of Advanced Nursing, Umeå University, Umeå, Sweden

and ASTRID NORBERG, *RN, PhD*
Professor, Department of Advanced Nursing, Umeå University, Umeå, Sweden

Twenty enrolled nurses (ENs), 20 registered nurses (RNs) and 20 physicians working in intensive care in northern Sweden narrated 255 stories about their experience of being in ethically difficult care situations. The ENs' stories mainly concerned problems relating to relationship ethics, the stories narrated by the physicians mainly concerned problems relating to action ethics, while the RNs' stories gave equal attention to both kinds of problems. The most common theme of both the RNs' and the physicians' stories was that of too much treatment. An obvious similarity between the ENs, RNs and physicians was that they saw themselves as equally lacking in influence in ethically difficult care situations. The only apparent difference between the three groups, however, was that the ENs brought up relationship problems more often than the others. Thus, the differences between the RNs and the physicians were fewer than usually reported in the literature. This might be related to the specialization of intensive care.

Introduction

Caring for critically ill patients in an intensive care unit means that difficult ethical problems must be faced and dealt with. Decisions of vital importance to the patient often have to be taken instantly. Previous research has described ethical problems mainly concerning organ donation (e.g. Omery & Caswell 1988), how priorities should be made in the provision of care (e.g. Gerlach-Engborg *et al.* 1989; Munoz *et al.* 1989), as well as withholding and withdrawing treatment (e.g. Berggren *et al.* 1991; Gilmour & Rosenberg 1989).

Questions can be asked from an action ethics perspective, i.e. focusing on the choice of the right action, as well as from a relationship ethics perspective;

how people relate to each other in various situations (Lindseth 1992). Moral development has been described from the action ethics perspective of Kohlberg (1981) as an increased ability to reason in accordance with abstract and general ethical principles in a context-independent way. Vitz (1990) reasoned mainly from a relationship ethics perspective and described moral development as an increasing ability to use narrative thinking in a context-dependent way.

Another way of stating the difference between various approaches to ethics is to differentiate between the ethics of justice and the ethics of care (Ford & Lowery 1986). Puka (1991) said that the two perspectives presuppose each other; you must care in order to be fair and in order to care you must be fair.

The study

This study presupposes that the analysis of the stories about people in ethically difficult care situations reveals both action ethics as well as relationship ethics perspectives and that the relationship between action ethics and relationship ethics perspectives is complex. People can reflect on their choice of action, on the effect of their actions, on their relationships and on the effect of their relationships to other people.

The rationale behind the use of a narrative approach (MacIntyre 1985; Sarbin 1986) is that human experience is always understood within a whole, which gives it its meaning. This whole constitutes a story; we tell our story and we are also told as a story. When we narrate something, the lived story is the starting point of the told story. Narrating an experience means giving meaning to the experience. A story demonstrates the complex interplay between cognitive, emotional and conative elements (Locke 1983; Tappan 1990) and is believed to disclose some 'tacit' knowledge (Vitz 1990) and provide new insights.

It is difficult to study ethical reasoning in practice. Our values are part of our 'taken for granted' common sense, woven into our culture. Narrating situations can make us aware of the values that guide our thinking and acting. Thus narratives about ethically difficult care situations may disclose differences of perceptions, feelings, reasoning and actions.

Walker *et al.* (1991) found that registered nurses (RNs) and physicians in general medical service identified different kinds of ethical problems when caring for the same patients. The RNs, for example, identified more problems related to patients' and families' wishes, while physicians perceived problems related to quality of life and economic factors. When Udén *et al.* (1992) interviewed RNs and physicians in medical and oncological care in northern Norway, they found that these two groups narrated their experience of being in ethically difficult care episodes differently. RNs stressed care and reasoned in accordance with relationship ethics, while physicians stressed justice and reasoned in accordance with action ethics. The RNs disclosed a lot of moral outrage (see also Pike 1991) which was said to relate to their problems in communicating with the physicians.

Ethical reasoning among enrolled nurses (ENs) has been addressed in a study of several categories of caregivers in dementia care (e.g. Norberg *et al.* 1987) but the ENs were not described separately. No study has been found focusing on ethical reasoning among ENs.

The aim of this study was to illuminate ENs', RNs' and physicians' experience of being in ethically difficult care situations by comparing their stories.

Method

Setting

This study was performed in northern Sweden, where most hospitals are public and patients pay a fixed daily rate irrespective of the type of medical treatment or level of care. The personnel in intensive care units consist of ENs with two years of training at upper secondary school, RNs with three years of college training, and physicians with about seven years of university training and four to five years of specialist training work. The chief physician (anaesthetist) is legally responsible for medical care as well as nursing care. The everyday nursing is run by a ward sister. An EN works with practical nursing tasks, taking care of one or two patients, while an RN is responsible for one to four patients and also for one to four ENs.

Subjects

To find out if the experience of ethically difficult care situations varies depending on level of expertise, gender and professional role, a sample of ENs, RNs and physicians was selected from intensive care units at six different hospitals. The rationale behind the selection of interviewees from the three professional groups was the fact that previous research has shown that professionals on different levels of expertise (Corley & Selig 1992) and of different gender (Ford & Lowery 1986) narrate care episodes in different ways.

After the study has been approved by the Ethics Committee at the Medical Faculty, Umeå University, the medical head of each clinic was asked to select a less experienced person from each professional group, men as well as women. All but one RN agreed to participate in the study. She was replaced by another nurse. Five of each category – less experienced/more experienced female and male ENs ($n = 20$), RNs ($n = 20$) and physicians ($n = 20$) – were interviewed from October 1991 to September 1992. Their characteristics are shown in Table 10.1.

Table 10.1   Characteristics of interviewees ($n = 60$).

	ENs		RNs		Physicians	
	LE	ME	LE	ME	LE	ME
Interviewees	10	10	10	10	10	10
Mean age	28	38	28	41	36	46
Range	22–36	28–59	21–33	31–51	28–48	40–59
Years in intensive care	2	10	2	13	1	16
Range	0.2–8	2–25	0.4–5	5–22	0.1–5	5–27

LE = less experienced. ME = more experienced.

Interviews

A tape-recorded transcribed personal interview was performed. The interviewees were asked to narrate an ethically problematic care episode that they had experienced at the ward, i.e. a situation where they felt uncertain about what was the good and/or right thing to do. Only additional narrative questions were asked (e.g. When? What next? Who? How did you feel?) to clarify the circumstances described in the stories (see also Mishler 1986).

All interviewees related more than one care episode. All in all there were 255 stories: 92 stories narrated by ENs, 80 stories narrated by RNs and 83 narrated by physicians (Table 10.2). When the narrative had ended, the interviewee was asked about his or her reflections on the episode that she/he had narrated. The interviews lasted from 20 to 70 minutes (mode = 30).

Table 10.2   Number of narrated stories.

	ENs		RNs		Physicians	
	LE	ME	LE	ME	LE	ME
Number of care episodes	46	46	40	40	35	48
Total 255	92		80		83	

LE = less experienced. ME = more experienced.

Interpretation of interviews

A phenomenological–hermeneutic analysis inspired by the philosophy of Ricoeur (1976, 1984; Brown *et al.* 1989) was performed. Each interview was regarded as a text. The stories about the interviewees being in an ethically difficult care situation were extracted and analysed in steps. First, a naïve reading of each interview was performed in order to acquire a sense of the whole. Second, a structural analysis with narrative categories was made. In accordance with this approach used in the study, the third step should be to interpret each interview seen as a whole again, taking the naïve reading and the structural analysis into account. This step will be performed later on. Because of the great number of stories ($n = 225$) it was decided to make an overview of the narrative structure of the stories before more detailed analyses were performed. In this chapter this overview is presented. Summaries of typical stories illustrate the material.

Structural analysis

Main plot

The plot of a narrative arranges the various events into a whole (Polkinghorne 1988). Therefore, the main content of each story was characterized and it was stated whether the action aspect or the relationship aspect dominated. The plot dominating a story was labelled 'main plot'. In order to make the main plot explicit the following questions were asked during the analysis: what choice of action does the story represent (action ethics); what does the story tell about the relationships between the actors (relationship ethics).

Outcome

In order to define the outcome of the story the following question was asked: how does the story end? The results were then classified from the interviewees' point of view into positive, negative or neutral outcomes.

Findings

Main plot

Fifty-four per cent of the stories dealt mainly with relationship problems, while 46% mainly concerned the choice of action. When the three professional groups were compared, without taking gender and level of expertise into account, the following pattern emerged (Fig. 10.1). Relationship problems were seen to be the main plot of the ENs' stories; relationship problems and problems to find the right action were brought up in equal proportions by the RNs. The physicians mostly brought up problems relating to the choice of action. The content of the main plots of the stories differed in the three professional groups. Six types of main plots were found; relationship to patients, to the patients' families and to other professionals (relationship problems), and withdrawing treatment, withholding treatment and too much treatment (problems concerning the choice of action).

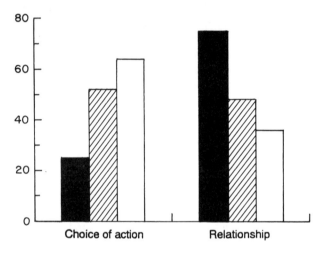

Fig. 10.1 Differences between the professional groups concerning relationship problems or the choice of action: graph of distribution of categories in percentages. ■ = EN; ▨ = RN; □ = physician.

When the main plots of the stories of the three groups investigated were compared, the following pattern emerged (Fig. 10.2). Too much treatment was the most common problem for the physicians and RNs. In addition, these two groups of professionals often brought up nearly the same aspect of the problem; the physicians related situations where they had not had enough influence to convince the physicians of the 'mother clinic', of the need to withdraw or withhold certain medical treatment. The RNs narrated care episodes where they had been ashamed of the care provided, but where they had not had enough courage or influence to change things the way they wanted, especially vis-à-vis the physician.

A physician narrated:

'This episode concerned a woman with some sort of cancer, the outcome of which was known to be very poor. She had been given a very aggressive anticancer treatment. She had nearly no thrombocytes and developed ARDS (adult respiratory distress syndrome). She was placed in a

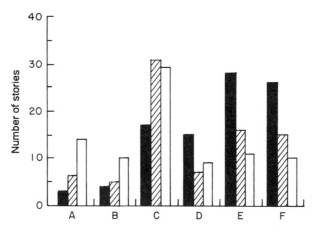

Fig. 10.2 The number of ENs', RNs' and physicians' stories with different main plots. ■ = EN; ▨ = RN; □ = physician. A = withhold treatment; B = withdraw treatment; C = too much treatment; D = relation professions; E = relation patients' families; F = relation patients.

respirator because the internist was of the opinion that the ARDS was a side-effect of the anticancer treatment and as soon as that had been overcome she would recover. Her lungs became so inelastic, though, that the respirator did not manage to press oxygen into them. The internist wanted to start an ECLA-treatment (to extract carbon dioxide and to supply the blood outside the body with oxygen). There have been no reports in medical literature about anyone suffering from this type of illness surviving such treatment. Besides, the patient would bleed to death when the cannulae was inserted into her vascular. It was impossible for me to convince the internist to withhold the ECLA-treatment and let her die in peace and with dignity with her family around her. A lot of specialists were called for and nearly all resources available at the hospital were involved. The patient died as soon as the surgeon started to operate. The surgeon was shocked and so were all the other people involved. Have human beings no right to die in peace? Do we allow technical science to provide absurd medical treatment? The next morning I went to the head of this clinic and asked him frankly, "Has an anaesthetist no right to decide about the treatment of a patient?" He answered: "Actually no, we are a service institution".'

An RN narrated:

'A man with leukaemia had been given several anti-cancer treatments but his cancer had not been cured. One night he suddenly became worse and I thought he was dying. However, instead of accepting this and letting him die with dignity, a very aggressive anticancer treatment was administered.

The intravenous catheter suddenly stopped functioning, so we tried to insert a new one but failed. We pricked him all over and he was grunting and groaning all the time, because he dreaded those tubes more than anything else. All of us knew that, but now the physicians ignored it and we continued this treatment until he died. I felt so sorry for him having to die like that and I felt so ashamed about the care provided because it violated his integrity.'

Mostly, the main plot of the ENs' stories concerned the relationship with patients' families. Families can visit their loved ones whenever they like. Having them sitting in the ward together with the patient most of the day, worried and emotionally affected, is often a difficult situation for ENs to handle. Problems concerning the relationships between patients, patients' families and professionals, as well as problems concerning information, decision making and treatment, become evident in the relationship between ENs and patients' families; the ENs sometimes feel like scapegoats and are made responsible for actions they can neither understand nor influence.
An EN narrated:

'Team-work among professionals helps me emotionally in difficult situations. ENs depend on other professionals because we are not in a position to make decisions on our own. I realized that once, when I was caring for a badly injured little child. Caring for children in this unit is usually very nice. Everyone comes into the ward to babble with the baby and talk to its parents. But this time everything was different, because the parents had caused the injury by battering the baby. It was a traumatic experience for me. I could not talk to the parents without resentment and I could not possibly understand how anyone could do such a dreadful thing to their own child. The RN in charge that day was new and completely unknown to me and so was the physician. They hardly entered the room at all, so I knew very little about what went on or what had been planned for the child. I found myself right in the middle of it, in the middle of the trying situation, but I felt like an outsider. I could hardly manage the situation by myself. I felt so vulnerable and lonely and missed the co-operation with other professionals.'

Stories about the relationship to parents included a variety of episodes, from moments of sorrow when someone, for example, had to tell a patient, 'Your family died in that car accident' or 'You are tetraplegic', to moments of happiness, as when an unconscious patient came to. The relationship to patients also concerned other issues: for instance, how to face patients' suffering, how to interpret the wishes of unconscious patients, and how to prevent moral outrage and repression.

Outcome of the stories

Sixty-seven per cent of the 255 stories had a negative outcome; (65% for the RNs', 69% for the physicians' and 67% for the ENs' stories). Four per cent of the stories had positive outcomes and 60% were negative all through, while 7% started in a positive way and ended negatively and 23% started negatively and ended positively. The remaining 6% of the stories were neutral.

An example of a typical story with a positive outcome narrated by an EN follows:

'A "long-stay" patient was taken down as a "no CPR" (no cardio-pulmonary resuscitation) after several months of intensive care without success. I felt that the "no CPR" wasn't right in his particular case. He wasn't very old and he had been very fit before the operation when the complications started. One day his heart actually stopped and I realized that I couldn't just stand there witnessing his dying, doing nothing. So I pressed the alarm and started to try to bring him back to life. Other professionals arrived and continued my job successfully. When everything was over I got frightened and asked myself: "What have I done? Was this the right thing to do?" Then the ward sister came and supported me by assuring me that I had done very well. The physician grumbled though: "This was a 'no CPR-patient'..." but nothing more was said about it. Some months later the patient was discharged and could return to his home. He is now doing very well and I'm so pleased! I think we need better co-operation between all groups of professionals before decisions about the level of treatment of critically ill patients can be made.'

An example of a typical story with a negative outcome narrated by an RN follows:

'A woman arrived at the hospital with a pain in her chest. We suspected myocardial infarction so she was observed during the night, but ECG did not show the pattern typical for this kind of illness, nor did her blood tests. I felt that this was no cardiac failure. The next morning the anaesthetist arrived asking the internist angrily, "*Why* hasn't the patient been given Actilyse?" The internist felt ashamed and, after some arguing, the angry and upset internist prescribed Actilyse. I reacted, but I said nothing. After the administering of drugs the patient suffered serious complications! This was no myocardial infarction, but an injury in the vertebral column! Why didn't I say something? I felt so guilty! Sometimes we must challenge the prestige of other professionals. We must talk to wake them up, and make them use their common sense.'

The turning point of the stories that changed from the negative to the positive or vice versa was often regarded as connected with the communication or lack of communication between the interacting parties.

An RN's story:

'An old dying man was prescribed more blood. I said to the physician in charge, "Come with me and take a look at the patient! Sit down here by his bed. There was a horrible and rotten smell in there. Now, look when I clean his mouth!" Mucous came out and the physician said, "I think we'll wait with the blood." When you come into the close perspective of the patient you often change your mind.'

A physician's story:

'There was a man with a severe vascular disease. In spite of this he was operated on for the rupture of a scar. He got thrombosis and all the complications you can imagine. He was treated in the intensive care unit week after week. Everyone involved suffered. There was no hope for him, and still the treatment continued. It was not possible nor legal to bring up the matter of treatment for discussion. One weekend an internist arrived asking us to reconsider our decision to continue the haemodialysis on our patient. She said that the resources were limited and that patients with some chance to survive needed these resources better. So we were forced to discuss the matter and suddenly it was quite all right to talk about it. We found that the internist was quite right, but the strange thing was that we needed the help of an internist to start such a reflective discussion.'

Discussion

Twenty ENs, 20 RNs and 20 physicians in intensive care units narrated their being in ethically difficult care situations. An analysis of the 255 stories revealed that there were fewer differences between the stories as narrated by RNs and physicians than could be expected judging from previous research. The most unexpected finding was that so many of the RNs' stories concerned the choice of action, because previous papers have claimed that RNs are usually concerned with relationships (e.g. Cooper 1990; Udén *et al.* 1992). One explanation might be that RNs respond to the decisions, or lack of decisions, of physicians as to what actions to take or withhold. Thus, physicians can be seen as the 'authors' of the RNs' stories. This may be particularly evident in intensive care, where medical treatment is so dominant.

Previous research has found differences between RNs' ethical reasoning in different settings (Jansson & Norberg 1989, 1992). In intensive care the RNs have to implement medical decisions to a considerable extent and therefore they must consult physicians several times a day. So it seems reasonable that they regard the choice of the level of treatment as problematic. The stories showed the problems RNs face when the treatment violates the integrity of the patient. The fact that the main plot of the RNs' stories so often dealt with the choice of action does not necessarily mean that RNs are not deeply concerned about relationships. Our analysis focused only on the main plot of the stories. The integration of action ethics and relation ethics in the narratives will be reported elsewhere.

The only apparent differences found were that ENs brought up relationship problems more often than the others. This may be a consequence of the organization of care. An EN sits alone with the patient and his/her family and cannot take part in, or listen to, the discussions on treatment among RNs and physicians. ENs try very hard to make the most of a situation and to come close to patients and their families, because a good relationship to them is a prerequisite to manage the implementation of nursing tasks. Thus it seems natural that relationship problems are important to them, especially as they interact with people in traumatic crises. The fact that ENs spend so much time with patients and patients' families makes it more difficult for them to distance themselves from relationship problems (see Duff 1987 about 'distant' versus 'close-up' ethics).

Too much treatment

The analysis of the 255 stories revealed that too much treatment was a big problem for the RNs and physicians involved. The way they narrated this indicated that many of them regretted that patients have too much treatment as well as meaningless treatment. They regarded this as an ethical dilemma associated with the decision to withhold and withdraw treatment. This theme has been widely discussed in medical literature and intensive care, in Sweden (e.g. Berggren *et al.* 1991) and in other countries (e.g. Bone *et al.* 1990). An obvious similarity between the ENs, RNs and physicians was that they saw themselves as lacking in influence in ethically difficult care situations. The stories, however, often showed that they concealed this feeling from their colleagues.

The interviewees' main problem did not always seem to be to decide what was the right and good thing to do, but rather how to do the right and good thing. This finding is similar to that of Udén *et al.* (1992), who found that RNs often related stories about situations where they knew how to act but were stopped by physicians. Pike (1991) also described ethical problems originating in communication difficulties between RNs and physicians. They said that with improved collaboration moral outrage will decrease.

Narrating ethically difficult care episodes is one way to make our personal values explicit and open to reflection and discussion. Thus, discussing ethical matters means disclosing more aspects of problematic situations, improving our ability to perceive the complex patterns of care episodes.

Acknowledgements

The authors would like to thank the interviewees who participated in the study. Ms Åsa Sundh and Mr Folke Rhedin Umeå, who revised the English.

References

Berggren, L., Olsson, J. & Sjökvist, P. (1991) Intensive care in the terminal phase of life: ethical considerations (Swedish). *Läkartidningen*, **88**(20–7), 2368–70.

Bone, R.C., Rackow, E.C. & Weg, J.G. (1990) Ethical and moral guidelines for the initiation, continuation, and withdrawal of intensive care: an ACCP-SCCM consensus panel. *Chest*, **97**(4), 949–58.

Brown, L.M., Tappan, M.B., Gilligan, C., Miller, B.A. & Argyris, D.E. (1989) Reading for self and moral voice: a method for interpreting narratives of real-life moral conflict and choice. In *Entering the Circle. Hermeneutic Investigation in Psychology* (Eds M.J. Packer & R.B. Addison), pp. 141–64, 306–9. State University of New York Press, Albany.

Cooper, M.C. (1990) Reconceptualizing nursing ethics. *Scholarly Inquiry for Nursing Practice: An International Journal*, **4**(3), 209–18.

Corley, M. & Selig, P. (1992) Nurse moral reasoning using the nursing dilemma test. *Western Journal of Nursing Research*, **14**(3), 380–88.

Duff, R.S. (1987) 'Close-up' versus 'distant' ethics: deciding the care of infants with poor prognosis. *Seminars in Perinatology*, **11**(3), 244–53.

Ford, M.R. & Lowery, C.R. (1986) Gender differences in moral reasoning: a comparison of the use of justice and care orientations. *Journal of Personality and Social Psychology*, **50**(4), 777–83.

Gerlach-Engborg, P., Englund, M-L., Samuelsson, C. & Sandstedt, S. (1989) Elderly in intensive care: is it profitable for society? (Swedish) *Läkartidningen*, **86**(44), 3765–6.

Gilmour, J.M. & Rosenberg, P.J. (1989) Medicolegal considerations in the initiation and termination of resuscitation in Canada. *Canadian Medical Association Journal*, **140**(3), 279–88.

Jansson, L. & Norberg, A. (1989) Ethical reasoning concerning the feeding of terminally ill cancer patients. *Cancer Nursing*, **12**(6), 352–8.

Jansson, L. & Norberg, A. (1992) Ethical reasoning among registered nurses experienced in dementia care. Interviews concerning the feeding of severely demented patients. *Scandinavian Journal of Caring Sciences*, **6**(4), 219–27.

Kohlberg, L. (1981) *Essays on Moral Development, Vol. 1. The Philosophy of Moral Development.* Harper & Row, New York.

Lindseth, A. (1992) The role of caring in nursing ethics. In *Quality Development in Nursing Care. From Practice to Science* (Udén), pp. 97–106. Health Service Studies, No. 7, Linköping Collaborating Centre, Linköping.

Locke, D. (1983) Doing what comes morally. The relation between behaviour and stages of moral reasoning. *Human Development*, **26**(1), 11–25.

MacIntyre, A. (1985) *After Virtue. A Study in Moral Theory*, 2nd edn. Duckworth, London.

Mishler, E. (1986) *Research Interviewing. Context and Narrative.* Harvard University Press, London.

Munoz, E., Josephson, J., Tenenbaum, N., Goldstein, J., Shears, A.M. & Wise, L. (1989) Diagnosis-related groups, costs, and outcome for patients in the intensive care unit. *Heart & Lung*, **18**(6), 627–33.

Norberg, A., Asplund, K. & Waxman, H. (1987) Withdrawing feeding and withholding artificial nutrition from severely demented patients. Interviews with caregivers. *Western Journal of Nursing Research*, **9**(3), 348–56.

Omery, A. & Caswell, D. (1988) A nursing perspective of the ethical issues surrounding liver transplantation. *Heart & Lung*, **17**(6), 626–31.

Pike, A.W. (1991) Moral outrage and moral discourse in nurse–physician collaboration. *Journal of Professional Nursing*, **7**(6), 351 63.

Polkinghorne, D.E. (1988) *Narrative Knowing and the Human Sciences*. State University of New York Press, New York.

Puka, B. (1991) Interpretive experiments: probing the care–justice debate in moral development. *Human Development*, **34**(2), 61–80.

Ricoeur, P. (1976) *Interpretation Theory: Discourse and the Surplus of Meaning*. Texas Christian University Press, Fort Worth, Texas.

Ricoeur, P. (1984) The model of the text: meaningful action considered as a text. *Social Research*, **51**(1–2), 185–218.

Sarbin, T.R. (1986) The narrative as a root metaphor for psychology. In *Narrative Psychology. The Storied Nature of Human Conduct* (Ed. T.R. Sarbin), p. 3. Praeger Special Studies, New York.

Tappan, M.B. (1990) Hermeneutics and moral development: interpreting narrative representations of moral experience. *Developmental Review*, **10**(3), 239–65.

Udén, G., Norberg, A., Lindseth, A. & Marhaug, V. (1992) Ethical reasoning within nurses' and physicians' stories about care episodes. *Journal of Advanced Nursing*, **17**(9), 1028–34.

Vitz, P.C. (1990) The use of stories in moral development. New psychological reasons for an old education method. *American Psychologist*, **45**(6), 709–20.

Walker, R.M., Miles, S.H., Stocking, C.B. & Siegler, M. (1991) Physicians' and nurses' perceptions of ethics problems on general medical service. *Journal of General Internal Medicine*, **6**(5), 424–9.

Chapter 11
Spiritual aspects of nursing

LINDA A. ROSS, *BA, RGN, PhD*
Research Fellow, Department of Management and Social Sciences, Queen Margaret College, Edinburgh, Scotland

In this chapter the author relates how she initially became interested in spiritual care. A synopsis of a literature review is given in which the spiritual dimension is defined and evidence presented for its influence on health, wellbeing and quality of life. Spiritual care is also presented as part of the nurse's role. However, it is acknowledged that there is a lack of guidelines for the practice of spiritual care. A conceptual framework for the latter is, therefore, proposed by the author. As little is currently known about how nurses perceive the spiritual dimension and their role in spiritual care, the findings from a doctoral study, which examined these issues, are reported and discussed. The descriptive study was part of the author's PhD thesis (Waugh 1992).

Background to this study

In her clinical practice, the author observed that sometimes there are patients who do not appear to have much physically wrong with them but seem to give up the will to live and die. On the other hand, there are patients who, despite terrible diagnoses and prognoses, seem determined to pull through and do so. This led the author to question the influence of the will to live and the spiritual dimension in general on an individual's state of health/illness, wellbeing and quality of life. In order to explore these issues, the relevant literature was reviewed.

Review of the literature

A plethora of definitions of the spiritual dimension was identified. A definition by Renetzky (1979), however, seems to summarize all others. He defines the spiritual dimension in terms of its three component parts:

(1) The need to find meaning, purpose and fulfilment (MPF) in life, suffering and death.

(2) The need for hope/will to live.
(3) The need for belief and faith in self, others and God.

Support for the influence of the spiritual dimension on health, wellbeing and quality of life was found and is presented here by considering each component of the above definition in turn, as available in the literature.

Meaning, purpose and fulfilment

According to Yura & Walsh (1982): 'the greatest task of human kind is to determine the meaning of life.' Stoll (cited in Rinear & Buys 1985) states: 'It has been said that man needs reasons for living and if there are none he begins to die.' Furthermore, Frankl & Travelbee (cited in Dickinson 1975), together with many other authors, regard the need for meaning as a universal trait that is essential to life itself (Autton 1980; Colliton 1981).

Frankl (1959) and Burnard (1989) assert that, when there is an inability to invest life with meaning, spiritual distress is the outcome and is characterized by feelings of emptiness and despair. A number of research studies highlight the importance of meaning in life for health and wellbeing. Simsen (1985) found that medical and surgical patients demonstrated a need to find meaning, in their illness and hospitalization. Although based on a small sample of 45 patients in a specific area of England, the study indicates that, within the sample, search for meaning was a significant experience for these patients. This is one of the few British studies addressing spirituality.

Kobassa (cited in Martin & Carlson 1988) reported fewer negative stress symptoms in individuals who were committed to and found meaning in their work. Detailed information about the method used, however, was not available and hence the validity and reliability of the results are not clear. Frankl (1959) and Antonovsky (1979), in their observations of holocaust victims, reported survival, minimal psychological damage and even strengthening of character in those who had managed to maintain a sense of meaning and purpose in their lives throughout their ordeal.

Renetzky (1979) sought to discover the relationship between MPF and spiritual well-being and found that as MPF increased so did the role of religion and the degree of healthy self-love, while the void or feeling of emptiness decreased. The findings of this single study conducted in the USA cannot be generalized. However, the study supports the supposition that as MPF increases so does the level of spiritual wellbeing and consequently quality of life and health.

To summarize this section, it would appear that the quest for MPF in life is fundamental to the attainment of an optimum state of health, wellbeing and quality of life.

Hope/will to live

Hope has been regarded as a major motivator of behaviour, acting as a powerful life force, producing vitality and liveliness in life (Dubree & Vogelpohl 1980). Widespread documentation gives evidence of the fact that without hope, death can result. For instance, both animal and human studies show that prolonged and repeated encounters with situations which, although not life threatening, are unavoidable and in which the outcome is independent of all voluntary responding, produce hopelessness. The end product of this is frequently death. Such instances include voodoo death (Bettleheim *et al.*, cited in Seligman 1974) and concentration camp experiences (Frankl 1959). Furthermore, although a causal link is difficult to identify, Blenkner (cited in Renetzky 1979) noted higher mortality rates in elderly people who had been involuntarily institutionalized. It is because of its often drastic effects that helplessness/hopelessness has been appropriately termed 'passive suicide' (Limandri & Boyle 1978).

The importance of hope to life can be seen not only in death caused by its absence, but also in healing produced by its abundance. Evidence for the positive effects of hope can be seen in clinicians' observations of clients over a number of years. For instance, both Renetzky (1979) and Swaim (1962) reported that the greater the will to live, the greater the chance their clients had of overcoming illness.

A different type of evidence which reports non-verifiable events illustrates the positive effects of hope; for example, Tari (1978) and Gardner (1983) document numerous instances of miraculous events (e.g. healing of the deaf and blind, raising of the dead) where hope and also faith in God were central. These instances are hardly surprising if, as McGee (1984) states, the degree of hope is related to the perception of the individual. The bigger one's concept of God, the more things become possible and obtainable.

It is in recognition of the importance of hope that Dominian (1983), a psychiatrist, acknowledged that medical prognosis cannot be established on the basis of scientific data alone, but must be made in conjunction with the hope displayed by the patient. It would appear, therefore, that hope or a will to live is vital to life itself.

Belief and faith in self, others and God

After over 30 years of working as a sociologist, Renetzky (1979) reported his observation that, as an individual's belief in themselves and others increases, so does their will to live. Furthermore, this latter aspect, together with MPF and spiritual wellbeing, was increased to a significantly greater degree when belief in God also existed. Consequently, there was virtual extinguishing of the 'void'.

Other studies have indicated the influence of belief and faith on health. O'Brien (1982) noted that patients who had a positive religious perspective on life adapted more readily to the stress of haemodialysis. Martin & Carlson (1988) report the findings of two studies, by Carlson *et al.* in 1986 and by Byrd in 1984, which indicated the therapeutic effect of faith in reducing anger, anxiety, pulmonary oedema and the need for antibiotic therapy, and intubation, respectively. However, Martin & Carlson (1988) question these findings given the biased samples used and absence of tests to determine statistical significance.

Although further research is indicated to test these observations, it would appear that the optimum state of health, quality of life or wellbeing can best be attained when MPF in life, a will to live and belief and faith in self, others and God exist.

Spiritual care – a role for nurses?

Given the apparent influence of the spiritual dimension on health, wellbeing and quality of life, together with the fact that the function of nursing, according to the International Council of Nurses (ICN 1973) is to, 'promote health, to prevent illness, to restore health and to alleviate suffering', it would seem that spiritual care should be part of the nurse's role. To explore this further the nursing literature was reviewed, and it was found that codes of conduct, models of nursing and guidelines for nurse education, at both national and international levels, advocated that nurses should be giving spiritual care.

Codes of conduct

The United Kingdom Central Council for Nursing, Midwifery and Health Visiting (UKCC 1984) states that it is the duty of the nurse to: 'Take account of the customs, values and spiritual beliefs of patient/clients'. Furthermore, according to the ICN (1973): 'The nurse, in providing care, promotes an environment in which the values, customs and spiritual beliefs of the individual are respected.

Models of nursing

Models include consideration of the spiritual dimension either directly (Henderson 1977; Watson cited in Riehl-Sisca 1989) or by ascribing to the individual's wholeness (Weidenbach cited in Fitzpatrick & Whall 1983; Rogers cited in Riehl-Sisca 1989) and search for meaning (Fitzpatrick's Rhythm Model cited in Fitzpatrick & Whall 1983).

Guidelines for nurse education

Both British and international guidelines for nurse education indicate that spiritual care should be taught to nurses. For instance, in preparation for Project 2000 (UKCC 1986) it has been recommended that nurse education should:

'provide opportunities to enable the student to ... acquire the competencies required to: xiv) identify ... spiritual needs of the patient or client, devise a plan of care, contribute to its implementation and evaluation by demonstrating an appreciation and practice of principles of a problem solving approach.'

Furthermore, the ICN (1973) which, as stated previously, includes spiritual care in its code for nurses, considers that the code:

'will have meaning only if it becomes a living document applied to the realities of human behaviour in a changing society [and that] In order to achieve its purpose the code must be ... put before and be continuously available to students ... throughout their study and work lives.'

In conclusion, having examined codes of conduct, models of nursing and guidelines for nurse education, it is evident that spiritual care should be a nursing responsibility and not an optional extra. However, it would seem that there is a lack of guidelines for the practice of spiritual care, as indicated by the:

(1) Lack of a generally agreed definition of 'spiritual'.
(2) Lack of literature specifically on spiritual care.
(3) Apparent lack of attention credited to spiritual issues in nurses' education programmes.
(4) Lack of research.
(5) Lack of a conceptual/theoretical framework for spiritual care in nursing.

Proposed conceptual framework for spiritual care emerging from the literature

If nurses are to be expected to give spiritual care it is imperative that they have a conceptual framework to guide their practice. One such framework has been suggested by the author (Fig. 11.1) and is explained below.

An individual entering hospital will do so with particular spiritual needs. Whether or not these needs are met may determine the speed and extent of his/her recovery, and the level of spiritual wellbeing and quality of life experienced. It is important, therefore, that patients receive the necessary help to meet their spiritual needs.

One way of ensuring that patients' spiritual needs are met is by using the

The patient's spiritual state   Giving spiritual care
                                                 using the nursing process

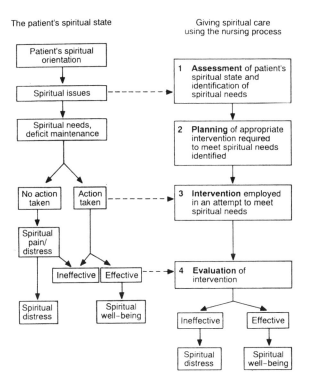

Fig. 11.1   A proposed conceptual framework for giving spiritual care using the nursing process.

nursing process as the mechanism to deliver systematic individualized spiritual care (Kratz 1979; Marriner 1983). This will involve identifying the patient's spiritual needs through conducting a spiritual assessment, planning and implementing the appropriate interventions to meet these needs, and evaluating the extent to which these interventions have been successful. At the outset this seems fairly simple. However, on closer examination it would appear that in order for each stage of the nursing process to be enacted, it will be necessary to have the knowledge outlined in Table 11.1.

Currently this knowledge is lacking. If nurses should be giving spiritual care, not only do they lack the knowledge to enable them to do so, but little is known about how they perceive their role in spiritual care.

Exploratory study

An exploratory, descriptive study was therefore designed to answer the following research questions:

(1) How do nurses perceive spiritual need and spiritual care and report to give the latter in practice?
(2) What factors appear to influence the spiritual care given to patients?

Table 11.1   Knowledge required in order for spiritual care to be given.

Stage of nursing process	Knowledge required
Assessment	What spiritual needs are. How they can be recognized (i.e. indicators of spiritual distress).
Planning and intervention	What might be appropriate interventions for the meeting of these needs.
Evaluation	What factors would indicate that the needs had been met (i.e. spiritual wellbeing indicators).

Results

Each question is addressed in turn and the results presented.

(1) Nurses' perceptions of spiritual need and spiritual care and their reports of how they gave that care

This question was answered by posing a number of sub-questions:

What do nurses understand by spiritual need?
Do nurses identify patients' spiritual needs?
How do nurses identify patients' spiritual needs?
How do nurses respond to patients' spiritual needs?
Who do nurses consider to be responsible for responding to patients' spiritual needs?
How do nurses evaluate the care given?

Staff nurses and charge nurses working full-time day and night duty on 'care of the elderly' wards in NHS hospitals in 12 Health Boards within Scotland were the respondents for the study. Having gained ethical approval, a purpose designed postal questionnaire was distributed to the population ($n = 1170$). Using a series of reminder letters, a 67.8% response rate was achieved. Closed and open questions were analysed with the help of the Statistical Package for the Social Sciences (SPSS) and the 'Ethnograph' (Seidel *et al.* 1988). The results are based on 685 usable responses and are presented below.

What do nurses understand by spiritual need?

Table 11.2 shows that, collectively as a group, nurses' definitions of spiritual need covered all aspects of the spiritual dimension definition outlined earlier. Also, the highest proportion of nurses defined spiritual need in terms of the need for belief and faith, this category being predominantly concerned with

Table 11.2 Nurses' definitions of spiritual need.

Definition	No. and % of nurses giving each response	
	No.	%
(1) Need for meaning, purpose and fulfilment	64	9.9
(2) Need to give and receive love and forgiveness	91	14.1
(3) Need for hope and creativity	23	3.6
(4) Need for belief and faith	221	34.1
(5) Need for peace and comfort	158	24.4
(6) Miscellaneous	90	13.9
Did not answer the question	38	

religious aspects. Thus it would seem that there is a tendency for nurses to view spiritual needs in religious terms.

Do nurses identify patients' spiritual needs?

It would appear that the majority of nurses identified patients' spiritual needs (Table 11.3). However, nurses were only asked if they had done so at some point in their practice. Therefore, there is no indication of the frequency with which they did so.

Table 11.3 Nurses' reports of whether or not they had identified a spiritual need.

Had identified a spiritual need	No. and % of nurses giving each response	
	No.	%
(1) Yes	503	76.8
(2) No	152	23.2
Did not answer the question	30	

How do nurses identify patients' spiritual needs?

Table 11.4 illustrates that nurses used a variety of indicators in identifying patients' spiritual needs. Through further breakdown of the categories it emerged that in 70% of cases spiritual needs were recognized through non-verbal means of communication. This finding suggests that spiritual needs are perhaps more subtle and more difficult to identify than some other needs and that whether or not they are identified may depend on the sensitivity of the nurse.

Table 11.4 Indicators nurses stated they used in recognizing patients' spiritual needs.

Indicators	No. and % of nurses giving each response	
	No.	%
(1) The need was expressed by the patient verbally or non-verbally	155	31.4
(2) The need was observed in other ways by the nurse	111	22.5
(3) Distress displayed by the patient	125	25.3
(4) State of helplessness displayed by the patient	47	9.5
(5) Patient unable to come to terms with situation	49	9.9
(6) Positive characteristics displayed by the patient	7	1.4
Did not answer the question	191	

How do nurses respond to patients' spiritual needs?

Table 11.5 shows that, although some nurses were willing to be intimately involved in helping patients meet their spiritual needs, e.g. those who were prepared to 'be with' the patient, over half did not but rather chose to refer to someone else.

Table 11.5 Nurses' definitions of spiritual care and/or stated responses to patients' spiritual needs.

Definition/response	No. and % of nurses giving each response	
	No.	%
(1) Recognizing/respecting/meeting patients' spiritual needs	44	6.8
(2) Facilitating participation in religious rituals	43	6.7
(3) Communicating: listening/talking with	42	6.5
(4) Being with the patient: caring, supporting, showing empathy	121	18.8
(5) Promoting a sense of wellbeing	58	9.0
(6) Referring to others	333	51.6
(7) Expressed difficulty in defining or giving spiritual care	4	0.6
Did not answer the question	40	

Who do nurses consider to be responsible for responding to patients' spiritual needs?

As can be seen in Table 11.6, almost all nurses (93.7%) considered themselves to be responsible, to some extent, for responding to patients' spiritual needs. However, bearing in mind the previous finding that the majority responded by referring to someone else, it would appear that nurses would like to be involved in spiritual care, but it tends not to happen for whatever reason.

Table 11.6 People nurses considered to be responsible for responding to patients' spiritual needs.

Person	No. and % of nurses giving each response	
	No.	%
(1) Nurse alone	0	0
(2) Clergy alone	37	5.6
(3) No one	2	0.3
(4) Nurse plus clergy	485	73.5
(5) Other* (only in 0.4% of cases did nurses exclude themselves from this role)	136	20.6
Did not answer the question	25	

* Includes any combination of the following: anyone; those outside the health care team, e.g. family, friends; clergy plus those outside the health care team; nurse plus clergy plus those outside the health care team.

Furthermore, 10% of nurses said retrospectively that they would have responded differently to patients' spiritual needs and most would have referred to someone else. This finding suggests that some nurses may not give spiritual care because they feel inadequate about doing so.

How do nurses evaluate the care given?

Tables 11.7 and 11.8 show that the majority of nurses considered their interventions to have been effective, and they reached this decision mainly through recognizing non-verbal cues which were the opposite of those which had led them to identify the needs in the first place.

In summary, nurses seemed fairly good at assessing patients' spiritual needs and evaluating the care given, but felt less able to respond for whatever reason, possibly because of feelings of inadequacy.

Table 11.7 Nurses' evaluations of the effectiveness of responses made to patients' spiritual needs.

Efficacy	No. and % of nurses giving each response	
	No.	%
(1) Totally effective	146	29.2
(2) More effective than ineffective	276	55.2
(3) Do not know	55	11.0
(4) More ineffective than effective	17	3.4
(5) Totally ineffective	6	1.2
Did not answer the question	185	

Table 11.8 Indicators nurses stated they used in evaluating the effectiveness of responses to patients' spiritual needs.

Indicators	No. and % of nurses giving each response	
	No.	%
(1) Eustressing characteristics displayed by the patient	174	37.6
(2) Patient appeared brighter in mood	48	10.4
(3) Patient's ability to accept situation	35	7.6
(4) Patient confirmed that his/her need had been met	78	16.8
(5) Nurse felt that the need had been met (not necessarily confirmed by the patient)	46	9.9
(6) Nurse felt that the need was not met/not completely met	28	8.0
(7) Nurse expressed difficulty in assessing the effectiveness of his/her interventions	54	9.7
Did not answer the question	222	

(2) Factors which appeared to influence the spiritual care given

Hockey (1979) found that the care her sample of district nurses gave was not entirely dictated by patients' needs but by a variety of other factors, such as the personal characteristics of the nurse, the administrative framework within which she had to operate and characteristics of the patient. It seemed appropriate, therefore, to seek to identify factors which may have influenced the spiritual care nurses gave. This information was sought in two ways, by cross-tabulation and interviews.

Variables were cross-tabulated and four were found to be significantly associated with the identification of spiritual needs by nurses. These related to the grade and belief system of the nurse and the type of ward and geographical area in which she/he was working.

Grade

Charge nurses were more likely to identify spiritual needs than staff nurses. However, this finding could not be explained by their length of experience or age.

Belief system

Nurses claiming religious affiliation were more likely to identify spiritual needs than those claiming none.

Type of ward

Nurses working on varied wards (e.g. long-term care and geriatric medicine) were more likely to identify spiritual needs than those working on non-varied wards (e.g. long-term care only).

Geographical area

Nurses working in some health boards were more likely to identify spiritual needs than those working in others. These findings raise more questions than they answer.

Interviews

In order to identify possible reasons for the above associations and to further explore factors which may have influenced the spiritual care nurses gave, semistructured interviews were conducted with a sample of nurses.

Twelve nurses were selected on the basis of set criteria. Although generalizations could not be made and the sample was too small for statistical treatment, it was hoped that the more detailed information would give some clues to possible factors influencing the spiritual care given.

Results

Analysis of the interviews revealed that four main groups of factors appeared to influence the spiritual care nurses professed to give. These related to the patient, other professionals, the environment and the nurse, as shown in Fig. 11.2.

The patient

It seemed that any factors which interfered with nurse–patient communication, e.g. deafness and dementia, made it difficult for nurses to identify spiritual needs. Perhaps if there was a predominance of patients suffering from conditions such as dementia in long-term care wards, this could explain the previous finding that nurses employed on non-varied wards reported having identified fewer spiritual needs than those working on varied wards.

Other professionals

Spiritual care was sometimes hindered if the clergy were not available, if in the nurse's opinion they had not performed their job properly, or if there was a lack of communication between the two disciplines. This finding perhaps suggests the need for greater collaboration between nurses and clergy.

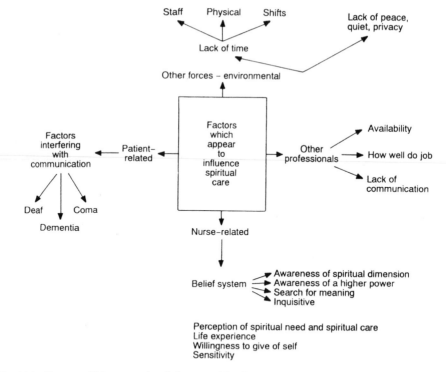

Fig. 11.2   Factors which appeared to influence spiritual care.

Environment

Nurses reported that lack of time, whether because of short staffing levels, pre-occupation with physical care or new shift patterns, interfered with the giving of spiritual care. This finding perhaps has implications for administrative decisions. Given the influence of the spiritual dimension on health, perhaps it would be more economically viable in the long term to ensure adequate staffing levels and to alter shift patterns to increase rather than reduce staff overlap. Nurses also reported that a lack of peace, quiet and privacy hindered them from giving spiritual care. This finding perhaps has implications for ward layout. It may be beneficial to have a quiet room set aside without a television where patients could have peace and quiet, or to have a rest hour as part of the ward routine.

The nurse

It appeared that spiritual care could be given on different levels. Some nurses were able to identify a broad range of spiritual needs and respond personally at a deep level. Others could identify a narrow range of needs only and responded at a more superficial level, i.e. by referring to someone else. The way in which nurses gave spiritual care seemed to be dependent on a number of personal characteristics. Nurses who gave spiritual care at a deep level demonstrated the following characteristics.

(1) They were aware of the spiritual dimension in their own lives. This finding suggests that the spiritual awareness of the nurse may be more important than the religious label she adopts in determining how she gives spiritual care (all interviewees were female).
(2) They had experienced crises which seemed to act as forces for growth, enabling them to become more self-actualized. This suggests that the life experience/maturity factor may be more important than the grade of the nurse in determining the care given by her.
(3) They were willing to give of themselves at a deep personal level, which may be associated with their life experience and spiritual awareness.
(4) They were particularly sensitive/perceptive people.

Nurses who gave spiritual care at a superficial level demonstrated all of the above characteristics to a lesser degree.

Conclusion

The spiritual dimension would appear to influence health, wellbeing and quality of life. From the literature it would seem that spiritual care is expected of nurses; however, guidelines for its practice are lacking. A conceptual framework is, therefore, proposed for giving spiritual care using the nursing process, but it is acknowledged that there is currently a lack of knowledge to enable it to be enacted.

The study sought to elicit nurses' perceptions of the spiritual dimension and spiritual care. The findings revealed that, within the sample, nurses seemed able to identify patients' spiritual needs and evaluate the care given, mainly through observing non-verbal cues displayed by the patient. However, they were less willing/able to respond personally to these needs.

Charge nurses claiming religious affiliation and working on varied wards in certain geographical locations seemed most likely to have identified spiritual needs. But, from the limited sample interviewed, it would seem that personal characteristics of the nurse are perhaps more important than these other factors in determining whether or not and how nurses gave spiritual care. Thus further research is required to clarify this possibility.

Furthermore, the unavailability and poor performance of other professionals, together with environmental factors and those interfering with nurse–patient communication, appeared to hinder the giving of spiritual care by nurses.

If nurses are to be expected to promote spiritual health and alleviate the spiritual suffering of patients, further research is required to provide them with the necessary guidelines. Thus patients could be helped to achieve their optimum state of health, wellbeing and quality of life, and in so doing nursing would have fulfilled its ultimate goal.

Acknowledgements

The author wishes to acknowledge her director of studies, Dr L. Hockey, and her supervisors, Miss E. Dove and Revd Dr D. Lyall, for their advice and support throughout the study, and Queen Margaret College, Edinburgh for providing the research studentship. Special thanks are also due to Dr L. Hockey for her helpful comments on the manuscript.

References

Antonovsky, A. (1979) *Health, Stress and Coping.* Jossey-Bass, San Francisco and London.
Autton, N. (1980) The hospital chaplain. *Nursing (Add-on Journal)*, **1**, 697–9.
Burnard, P. (1989) *Counselling Skills for Health Professionals.* Chapman and Hall, London.
Colliton, M.A. (1981) The spiritual dimension of nursing. In *Clinical Nursing: Pathophysiological and Psychosocial Approaches*, 12th edn (Eds I.L. Beland & J.Y. Passos), pp. 492–501. Macmillan, New York.
Dickinson, C. (1975) The search for spiritual meaning. *American Journal of Nursing*, **75**(10), 1789–93.
Dominian, J. (1983) Doctor as prophet. *British Medical Journal*, **287**(6409), 1925–7.
Dubree, M. & Vogelpohl, R. (1980) When hope dies so might the patient. *American Journal of Nursing*, **80**(11), 2046–9.
Fitzpatrick, J.J. & Whall, A.L. (1983) *Conceptual Models of Nursing: Analysis and Application.* Robert J. Brady, New Jersey.
Frankl, V.E. (1959) *Man's Search for Meaning.* Washington Square Press, Washington.
Gardner, R. (1983) Miracles of healing in Anglo-Celtic Northumbria as recorded by the Venerable Bede and his contemporaries: a reappraisal in the light of twentieth century experience. *British Medical Journal*, **287**(6409), 1927–33.
Henderson, V. (1977) *Basic Principles of Nursing Care.* ICN, Geneva.
Hockey, L. (1979) A study of district nursing. The development and progression of a long term research programme. Unpublished PhD thesis, City University, London.
ICN (1973) *Codes for Nurses. Ethical Concepts Applied to Nursing.* ICN, Geneva.
Kratz, C. (1979) *The Nursing Process.* Baillière Tindall, London.
Limandri, B.J. & Boyle, D.W. (1978) Instilling hope. *American Journal of Nursing*, **78**(1), 79–80.
McGhee, R.F. (1984) Hope: a factor influencing crisis resolution. *Advances in Nursing Science*, **6**(4), 34–44.
Marriner, A. (1983) *The Nursing Process. A Scientific Approach to Nursing Care*, 3rd edn. C.V. Mosby, St. Louis, Missouri.
Martin, J.E. & Carlson, C.R. (1988) Spiritual dimensions of health psychology. In: *Behaviour Therapy and Religion* (Eds W.R. Miller & J.E. Martin), pp. 57–110. Sage, Beverly Hills.
O'Brien, M.E. (1982) Religious faith and adjustment to long term haemodialysis. *Journal of Religion and Health*, **21**(1), 68.
Renetzky, L. (1979) The fourth dimension: applications to the social services. In *Spiritual Wellbeing: Sociological Perspectives* (Ed. D.O. Moberg), pp. 215–54. University Press of America, Washington.

Riehl-Sisca, J. (1989) *Conceptual Models for Nursing Practice*, 3rd edn. Appleton & Lange, Connecticut.

Rinear, E.E. & Buys, A.M. (1985) Spiritual and religious dimensions of psychiatric mental health nursing. In *Psychiatric Nursing in the Hospital and the Community*, 4th edn (Ed. A.W. Burgess), pp. 866–79). Prentice-Hall, Englewood Cliffs, New Jersey.

Seidel, J., Kjolseth, R. & Seymour, E. (1988) *The Ethnograph. A Program for the Computer-Assisted Analysis of Text-Based Data.* Qualis Research Associates, Colorado.

Seligman, M.E.P. (1974) Submissive death: giving up on life. *Psychology Today*, 7(12), 80–85.

Simsen, B.J. (1985) Spiritual needs and resources in illness and hospitalisation. Unpublished MSc thesis. University of Manchester.

Swaim, L. (1962) *Arthritis, Medicine and Spiritual Laws.* Chilton Book Company, Philadelphia.

Tari, M. (1978) *Like a Mighty Wind.* Kingsway, Eastbourne.

UKCC (1984) *Code of Professional Conduct for the Nurse, Midwife and Health Visitor*, 2nd edn. UKCC, London.

UKCC (1986) *Project 2000. A New Preparation for Practice.* UKCC, London.

Waugh, L.A. (1992) Spiritual aspects of nursing: a descriptive study of nurses' perceptions. Unpublished PhD thesis, Queen Margaret College, Edinburgh.

Yura, H. & Walsh, M. (1982) *Human Needs 2 and the Nursing Process.* Appleton-Century-Crofts, Norwalk, Connecticut.

Chapter 12
Discharge planning: issues and challenges for gerontological nursing. A critique of the literature

MARILYN F. JACKSON, *RN, BN, MEd*

Associate Professor, School of Nursing, University of Victoria, Victoria, British Columbia, Canada

Families are rapidly becoming unpaid givers of complex care. Using McKeehan & Coulton's systems model, this critique reviews the evolution of the structure and processes of discharge planning programmes. It explores three common assumptions: discharge planning programmes are cost-effective, allow for enhancement of patients' and families' quality of life, and ensure continuity of care between hospital and community. Funds are saved due to decreased lengths of initial hospital admissions and readmission rates. However, the cost of additional hospital and community resources is rarely considered. Little evidence supports the concept that discharge planning directly affects a patient's health status. Patients and families often do not perceive the same level of benefit from discharge planning as do health professionals. Several issues surrounding research methodologies used in the reviewed studies are identified. Of particular concern is the lack of qualitative research into patients' and families' experiences. The critique concludes with an exploration of ethical issues and challenges arising from increased emphasis on cost-effective discharge planning. These include patients' rights, provision of sufficient human, social and financial resources, improved hospital–community communications, and control over hospital-developed but community-implemented programmes.

Introduction

'[There is] a need for someone to help those who can become self-reliant, to obtain help for those who need it or else the medical care may fail of its good purpose. (Dr T. Loch, 1885, as cited in Blaylock & Cason 1992)

The frequently used phrase 'quicker and sicker' increasingly describes hospital discharge planning for the 1990s. Complex care required by many older discharged patients is rapidly becoming the responsibility of community-based health workers and unpaid family members (Johnson & Fethke 1985; George & Gwyther 1986; Hawe *et al.* 1986; Tierney & Closs 1993).

Discharge planning is a process and service where patient needs are identified and evaluated and assistance is given in preparing the patient to move from one level of care to another, hospital to home or hospital to another facility. It involves arranging that phase of care, whether it be self-care, care by family members, care by a paid health provider or a combination of options (American Nurses' Association 1975; Bristow *et al.* 1986; McKeehan 1981). Although much discharge planning is multidisciplinary, it is 'nurses [who] hold the key to assessing patient needs and to helping patients and families plan appropriately for transitions in care' (Rorden & Taft 1990).

Assumptions

A review of the literature determined that present discharge planning programmes are based upon three major assumptions such programmes are cost-effective; they provide a continuity of care which maintains if not improves the health status of discharged elderly patients, and they allow for the enhancement of patients' and families' quality of life. Using a model developed by McKeehan & Coulton (1985), this critique of the literature on discharge planning for acutely ill hospitalized elderly patients examines the reality of these assumptions. Finally, it explores the issues and challenges for nurses and other health professionals involved in geriatric hospital discharge programmes.

Literature sources

Literature sources for this critical review of discharge planning include papers and books on discharge planning for the acutely ill elderly patient, published between 1978 and 1992. Not included are unpublished works not readily available, such as unpublished dissertations, master's theses and conference proceedings. Print searches included cumulated index medicus, cumulated index to nursing and allied health literature, rehabilitation and physical medicine index, social science citation index, psychological abstracts and sociological abstracts. On-line computer searchers include Medline, CINAHL, Psyclit, Sociofile, and Ageline.

The structure, process and outcomes of discharge planning programmes (Fig. 12.1) are critically reviewed using a framework adapted from McKeehan & Coulton's model (1985). As a systems model, it allows for an

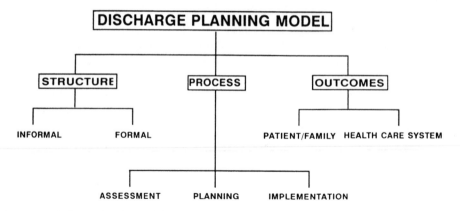

Fig. 12.1 Discharge planning model.

examination of discharge planning by viewing the relationship of its parts. It also permits an evaluation of the three-fold premise upon which discharge planning is based: cost-effectiveness for the health care system, continuity of care for patients and quality of life for patients and families.

Findings

Structure

In the McKeenan & Coulton model, a programme's structure is either informal or formal (Fig. 12.2). Until the late 1970s, much discharge planning

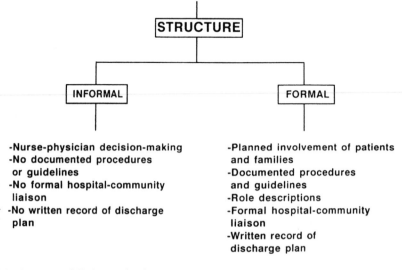

Fig. 12.2 Structure of discharge planning programmes.

was traditionally the responsibility of the staff nurse in consultation with the physician and perhaps a social worker. The patient and family were advised rather than consulted. As the demands by frail elderly people on hospital services increased, the term 'bed blocker' became part of hospital language.

By the 1980s there was a growing shift within universal health care systems towards a formal structure (Thliveris 1990). The UK was a leader in this movement towards specialization in the hospital care of elderly patients (Barker 1986). In the United States, the 1972 amendment to the American Social Security Act made discharge planning a specific requirement (McKeehan & Coulton 1985). By 1990, most discharge planning pro-grammes described in the literature use a formal structure with written programme policies, role descriptions, screening and assessment protocols, documentation requirements, methods for follow-up and programme eva-luation. However, what is described may not be happening; for example, Dugan & Mosel (1992), in a review of 101 American patient records, found that 46.2% had no documentation of any discharge planning.

Today, discharge planning programmes vary. They may have a one-person structure, usually a single designated nurse who consults with patients, families and other health professionals. Alternatively, they may consist of large multidisciplinary teams that meet on a regular basis (Borok *et al*. 1994). Haddock (1991), in her study of eight rural hospitals, reports that the more highly formalized the structure, the greater the provision of services and level of patient satisfaction. She also found that a follow-up programme such as a home visit gives reassurance to the patients and families who may be experiencing shock and anger at the reduced length of expected hospital stay.

Process

The discharge planning process involves assessment, planning and imple-mentation (Fig. 12.3).

Assessment – what

The five most common areas included in the assessment of high-risk older clients are cognitive, physical and social/financial status, environmental concerns, and access to formal and informal care. Of particular interest is a nursing staff's assessment of 'risk' and potentially 'risky discharges' (Mac-Millan 1994). Kane (1987) warns that information collected must be relevant to the medical treatment and rehabilitation of the patient. For example, endless amounts of data can be collected under the aegis of social assessment. Unfortunately, use of diverse assessment tools makes it difficult to compare the findings of research studies into discharge planning.

Elders who live with family caregivers have shorter hospitalization

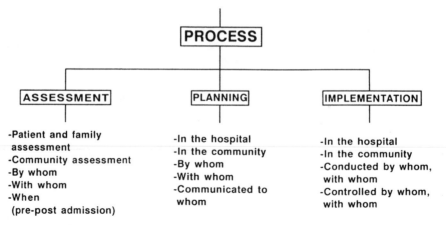

Fig. 12.3   Discharge planning process: assessment, planning and implementation.

(Skinner & Tennstedt, 1994). Thus, it is essential to assess family resources, coping strategies and informational needs (Corkery, 1989). To teach only the patient and not the family is dangerous, given that many older patients can only recall a small percentage of the information presented (Resseler 1991).

Some patients and families overestimate their ability to manage following discharge. An argument for home assessments is that they help determine the amount of stress and burden of caregiving with which a family can cope (Rosenblatt *et al.* 1986; Bull 1988). Unfortunately, home visits by patients and hospital staff, as described by MacDonald (1981), rarely occur in many North American settings.

Families need to know how to access help before the patient leaves the hospital. Nurses and others involved in discharge planning must be aware of available community resources and their appropriateness and acceptability to patients and families (Jacobs *et al.* 1985).

Assessment – when

There is agreement that planning for discharge must begin at least at the time of admission (Kane *et al.* 1983; Shine 1983; Cunningham 1984; Barker *et al.* 1985; Patterson 1986) or sooner when pre-admission screening is possible (Berkman *et al.* 1988). Yet, although critical care units admit many elderly patients, the majority of critical care nurses do not perceive discharge planning as part of their nursing mandate (Schlemmer 1989).

Proponents for pre-screening, including telephone screening, argue that pre-admission screening programmes facilitate the identification of psychosocial and home problems. They also allow for orchestration of appropriate post-hospital resources well in advance of any discharge (Berkman *et al.*

1988; Reardon *et al.* 1988). These authors argue that hospital assessments focus on the medical aspects of care and pay little attention to the functional status of elderly patients, such as ability to walk and climb stairs and to manage their medications (Warshaw *et al.* 1982; Rock *et al.* 1990).

Planning

Writers disagree on who should be responsible for discharge planning, who should be involved, and how and to whom discharge plans should be communicated. Planners vary from multidisciplinary discharge planning teams led by geriatricians (Berkman *et al.* 1983; Campion *et al.* 1983; Lichtenstein & Winograd 1984; Barker *et al.* 1985; Allen *et al.* 1986; Hogan *et al.* 1987; Pawlson 1988) to a single nurse, usually a geriatric clinical nurse specialist (Marchette & Holloman 1986; Kennedy *et al.* 1987; Markey & Igou 1987; Naylor 1990; Neary & Kitchen 1990). Two studies found that geriatric consultation teams had no significant impact on patient outcomes (Gayton *et al.* 1987; Saltz *et al.* 1988).

Some teams include community nurses and families, the rationale being that such arrangements bring a more holistic family-based approach to the assessment-planning process (Drew *et al.* 1988; Worth *et al.* 1994). Neary argues that such teams improve within-hospital and hospital–community communication (Neary & Kitchen 1990). Yet, as Edwards (1978) observes, if team activities become too structured, the flexibility needed to care for elderly people can be lost.

Medical literature views the physician as the team leader who is responsible for all aspects of discharge planning, acting as gatekeeper to all services. Other health professional literature views the physician as one member of the discharge planning team, with all members providing leadership in relation to their area of expertise and patient and family needs. Although most studies recommend a multidisciplinary approach, all literature reviewed on discharge planning was found to be discipline-specific.

The importance of the nurse and the nurse's attitude towards the rehabilitative potential of older patients cannot be over-emphasized (Heller *et al.* 1984; Johnson 1989). There is universal agreement that nurses play a major role in any plan, especially in educating clients and families about medications and other medical therapies (Markey & Igou 1987; Waters 1987a,b). Medication education by nurses is found to be as important to a successful outcome as arranging for a homemaker or a home care nurse (Felsenthal *et al.* 1986; MacGuire *et al.* 1987; Jackson 1989).

For a plan to be effective, it needs to be shared with those responsible for giving the care (Simmons 1986). Two communication formats stressed throughout the literature are informative *written* records and on-going case conferences. Both must be accessible to all persons involved in the care of the patient (Reichelt & Newcomb 1980; Waters 1987a). Several authors stress the complementary relationship between quality of communication between hospital staff, family and community personnel and patient outcomes (Cedar *et al.* 1980; Reichelt & Newcomb 1980; Agate 1985; Waters 1987a). Yet there is a paucity of studies on the effect of hospital–community communication on the implementation of a plan or on patient and family outcomes.

Generally a plan, to be successful, has to be based on the reality of the patient. There is a danger in planning too far in advance given the fragility of elderly patients, their potential for rapid change and the reality of regression in ability to function immediately after discharge (Wachtel *et al.* 1987). Thus the need for flexibility and opportunity to revise a discharge plan is paramount.

Implementation

Good working relations between staff, strong administration support and staff flexibility are essential factors for successful implementation of discharge planning programmes (Feather & Nichols 1985). Several studies indicate that the greater the level of patient and family involvement in the discharge planning process the more patients perceive themselves ready for discharge (Coulton *et al.* 1982; Jacobs *et al.* 1985; Simmons 1986). Also, successful outcomes occur more frequently when there is agreement between nurses' assessment and patients' perception of their own needs (Arenth & Mamon 1985; Schaefer *et al.* 1990).

There must be strong liaison between hospital and community services (Agate 1985). A simple liaison model involves person-to-person communication between individual hospital and community staff (Jowett & Armitage 1988). A more common model includes a community liaison nurse or social worker (Jowett & Armitage 1988; MacDonald 1981; Packard-Helie & Lancaster 1989). A third model reflects an integrated approach with the head nurse/unit manager acting in the liaison role (Jowett & Armitage 1988). Other options include joint management and staff education positions, and staff exchange programmes (Pellegrino & Buckley 1987; Pleasant 1991). No one approach has been proven to be more effective than another.

Anticipation of potential problems at home, use of home visits with family members present, and involvement of community nurses and occupational therapists in home assessments, assist in the successful implementation of a plan (MacDonald 1981; Buck & Mills 1988; Meeds & Pryor 1990); for example, the 'pharmacy of horrors' present in many home situations is well documented (Smith & Andrews 1983; Felsenthal *et al.* 1986; MacGuire *et al.* 1987).

Outcomes

A combination of effective geriatric rehabilitation matched with discharge placement appears to slow down the 'carousel of hospital admission and readmission' (Staff 1983; Smith *et al.* 1987; Dacher 1989). Unfortunately, there is a scarcity of published evaluations of discharge planning programmes to support this finding. Many authors address the need for more specific discharge criteria for measuring patient performance. In 1987, a panel of experts rated the overall quality of discharge planning in the USA as very poor (Fink *et al.* 1987). No similar non-American study could be found.

Most evaluations found are quantitative: decreases in number and frequency of patient care days, readmission rates, demand on post-discharge services, and scaling of patient and family satisfaction with the process (Schrager *et al.* 1978; Cable & Mayers 1983; Rubenstein *et al.* 1984; Marchette & Holloman 1986; Kennedy *et al.* 1987; Wachtel *et al.* 1987; Jackson 1990; Naylor 1990) (Fig. 12.4). Of interest are the reports on the effect of patient medication education prior to discharge. Such education was found to be a major influence in decreasing the numbers of hospital readmissions (Markey & Igou 1987; Naylor 1990).

Few qualitative studies of patients' and families' perceptions of their quality of life after discharge were found. Qualitative outcomes are stated tentatively, with researchers using such phrases as 'probably improved [their quality of life]', 'should improve [their quality of life]', 'inconsistent results as to [their quality of life]' (Applegate *et al.* 1983; Berkman *et al.* 1983; Cable & Mayers 1983; Teasdale *et al.* 1983; Davis *et al.* 1984; Victor & Vetter 1985; Waters 1987b; Saltz *et al.* 1988; Jackson 1989, 1990; Naylor 1990).

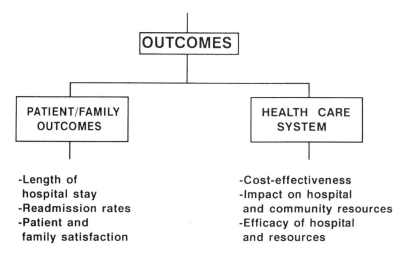

Fig. 12.4 Expected outcomes of discharge planning programmes.

Both individual and team approaches to discharge planning report positive outcomes, i.e. decreased patient care days and readmissions. There is no clear evidence that any one approach is best (Teasdale *et al.* 1983; Kennedy *et al.* 1987). There is some suggestion that a team approach encourages referrals to rehabilitation services with resultant increased patient ability to manage activities of daily living. Teams also appear to provide more information about community services (Berkman *et al.* 1983; Campion *et al.* 1983; Jackson 1984; Marchette & Holloman 1986; Williams *et al.* 1987).

Some studies report no significant impact of discharge planning on patient outcomes (Gayton *et al.* 1987; Naylor 1990). Such negative outcomes may be in part due to environmental factors such as hospital staff shortages (Graham & Livesley 1983). The finding of Caradoc-Davies *et al.* (1989) of lack of congruency between the staff's perception of the adequacy of the education and development of coping skills, and the clients' less favourable view is especially important for nurses. As Congdon (1994) reported in a study using a grounded theory design, the management of the 'incongruities of the discharge process [is] a struggle for patients and families'.

There is limited discussion in the literature of the need for patient advocacy. Dugan & Mosel (1992) found that persons living alone receive fewer community services than those who have a family member who can act as an advocate. Cost of community services may be a factor for single American seniors. However, there are important questions for health professionals working within universal health care systems. Are persons living alone disadvantaged when accessing community services? Do nurses and other caregivers need to be more active advocates for high-risk elders living alone?

Issues and challenges

Issues

It is difficult to compare the literature on discharge planning because of variations in basic research design, construct validity, populations targeted and outcomes measured (Schmitt *et al.* 1988; Hogan 1990). Differences in time frames make it difficult to compare results. For example, readmission rates for elderly patients range from 22% to 37% for periods ranging anywhere from six weeks to one year (Berkman & Abrams 1986; Weinberger *et al.* 1988).

Most studies are descriptive in nature, although some identify themselves as quasi-experimental research. Descriptive studies tend to support positive results, especially in the use of geriatric consultation teams. Quasi-experimental and experimental studies are split, 50% positive and 50% negative (Hogan *et al.* 1987; Hogan 1990). Although several used control and

experimental groups, only Allen *et al.* (1986) reported using a truly randomized population. Only one study used a double-blind approach (Kennedy *et
al.* 1987).

Data-collecting approaches include in-hospital interviews with patients,
families and staff, chart audits and follow-up visits to family/patient homes
and community-based nursing staff. There are no repeat studies. General-
ization of the results is not possible, given the small size of populations
studied. Follow-up of patients by hospital personnel is extremely limited at
best.

Challenges

Assumption – discharge planning programmes are cost-effective

Length of stay: There is evidence that discharge planning programmes are
cost-effective, especially when they result in decreased lengths of initial
hospital admissions and readmission rates (Schmitt *et al.* 1988; Naylor 1990;
Pleasant 1991). However, these calculations do not consider the expense of
additional community-based services and resource persons such as gerontological nurse specialists. Nor do they include the cost to families who are
rapidly becoming unpaid givers of complex care.

There is no clear evidence that discharge planning programmes have any
significant impact on the length of initial hospitalization. An American study
found that the earlier discharge planning is initiated after admission, the
shorter the length of stay, except for patients covered by Medicare (Farren
1991). Studies by Cable & Mayers (1983) and Naylor (1990) indicate that the
length of initial hospitalization may be more specific to the admitting diagnosis than to any discharge plan.

Availability of resources affects length of hospital stay. Most reported
studies are carried out in urban centres. Insufficient home care services,
especially in some rural and isolated settings (as in northern Canada), may
delay the discharge of some elderly persons to their own homes (Saltz *et al.*
1988).

Any decrease in readmission rates probably results in savings to the health
care system. In countries with universal health care systems, these savings are
a result of decreased need for additional hospital beds rather than from
empty beds on hospitals' acute care units.

Resource costs Any change in patient care and assessment causes an increase
in staff workload, especially on social workers and nurses (Feather & Nichols
1985). Neary & Kitchen (1990) found that novice nurses need additional
education to assess high-risk elderly patients and families. Additional staff

such as a geriatric nurse specialist increases salary costs (Neidlinger *et al.* 1987).

In addition, there are costs involved in getting a change in procedure accepted. As Wisendale reports, printed directories of community resources and educational programmes are easier to implement than a change to a team approach in assessing patients and planning their rehabilitation and discharge (Wisendale 1987). Yet few evaluations of discharge planning programmes include the effects of change, additional responsibilities on staff or the need for additional staff and staff education.

There is no evidence that the size or composition of a discharge planning team has any impact on patient outcomes. Interdisciplinary teams seem to result in fewer bureaucratic delays. However, the more inclusive the team is of other disciplines the greater the number of referrals to rehabilitation, nutrition and speech services. Such referrals may increase the length of hospital stay, thereby increasing the cost of patient care (Wertheimer & Kleinman 1990).

Increased sharing of information, community services and common data resources between hospitals and communities may provide financial and resource savings for health care systems. Such sharing would promote greater continuity of care to patients and family. Having older patients attend community-based day-centre programmes while still in hospital may be more cost-effective than developing a hospital-based rehabilitation programme (Nolan 1987; Morishita *et al.* 1989).

Assumption – discharge planning programmes provide a continuity of care which maintains if not improves the health status of discharged elderly patients

It is difficult to prove that discharge planning directly affects patients' health statuses. One reason is that poor patient outcomes are not always due to poor discharge planning. Readmissions may be due to several factors, including patient fragility and/or families' decreased ability to adapt to the constant physical and emotional stress of caregiving (Hunt 1980, Johnson & Fethke 1985, Andrews 1986, Berkman *et al.* 1987, Jackson 1989, 1990). New and unforeseeable problems or problems from the presence of chronic diseases with associated functional decline may occur. There may be non-compliance with a prescribed therapy. Families may under-assess their needs, such as need for special equipment in the home. Any one or a combination of such factors may cause an unexpected return to the hospital (Neary & Kitchen 1990, Wertheimer & Kleinman 1990, Trella 1991).

Age alone may be a contributing factor. The percentage of elderly people who need help with activities of daily living doubles with each successive decade up to age 84 years, and triples between ages 84 and 94 years (Almy & Health Policy Committee 1988). There is an increased incidence of chronic debilitating conditions with advanced age, with self-care deficits often disproportionate to the severity of the precipitating illness.

Assumption – discharge planning programmes allow for the enhancement of the quality of life for patients and families

Tierney *et al.* (1993), in a series of pre-and post-discharge interviews, identified three main problem areas: lack of preparation for discharge, inability to manage at home and limited provision of community services.

There is a lack of evidence that consultation occurs with patients and families about their concerns surrounding the discharge or about their own perceptions of needs. The inclusion of a family member on the discharge planning team does appear to increase caregiver understanding and satisfaction (Arenth & Mamon 1985).

Professionals insist that good liaison between hospital and community results in improved patient outcomes. Studies both support and contest this view. Caradoc-Davies *et al.* (1989) question whether patients or families perceive the same level of benefit as do health professions. Yet the Darlington [England] Project (Challis *et al.* 1991), using quantitative measures, reports a statistically significant improvement in the overall morale of elders discharged to the community compared to those discharged to continuing care institutions. Family caregivers of the project group experienced significantly less psychological stress. They reported preferring the stress of caring to the stress of guilt associated with the institutionalization of a family member (Challis *et al.* 1991).

Implications for further research

In spite of the growing amount of research on discharge planning, several questions remain unanswered; for example, what is the relationship between staff attitudes and patient outcomes, especially when a discharge planning programme results in increased workloads for already stressed nurses and social workers? Where are the standards against which the performance of a discharge planning programme can be measured? Does a hospital planning team's lack of authority over implementation of a discharge plan in the community negatively affect the outcome? For example, Ebrahim *et al.* (1987) showed that patients who attended out-patient rehabilitation following a stroke improved their functional ability. Yet only 42% of the 183 patients followed actually received any physio or occupational therapy after their discharge.

Is a geriatric consultant as effective as a geriatric team? This is especially important for smaller centres when a team approach is not a realistic option.

Does a team approach lead to increased number of diagnoses and additional costs or to lower levels of needed care with resultant savings over the longer term?

Client satisfaction is upheld in the health status literature as an appropriate variable. Yet there is a lack of qualitative studies into quality of life issues for patients and their families. There need to be evaluation studies that match groups of patients and families on a broader basis than diagnostic categories.

Ethical questions

There are many ethical questions surrounding discharge planning. Do patients have the right to deny having family as part of the planning process? Do older patients have the right to make what may be foolish and risky choices about where to live after their discharge (Dubler 1988)? Are there patients, given their health status and costs involved, who should not be in any discharge planning programme? What are appropriate screening criteria for use with such patients?

Discharge planning includes the placement of persons in long-term care facilities. A challenge to hospital staff is to ensure that the planning process distinguishes between coercion and choice, especially for elderly patients with diminished or fluctuating mental capacity.

Discharge planning places demands on all hospital and community resources: human, technical and financial. The more rigorous the search into ways of decreasing the cost of hospital care to older persons, the more rigorous must be the evaluation of discharge planning programmes for our vulnerable elderly populations.

References

Agate, J. (1985) Rehabilitation of the elderly patient: ways and means. *International Rehabilitation Medicine*, **7**, 109–15.

Allen, C.M., Becker, P.M., McVey, L.J. *et al.* (1986) A randomized, controlled clinical trial of a geriatric consultation team. *Journal of the American Medical Association*, **255**, 2617–21.

Almy, T.P. & Health Policy Committee, American College of Physicians (1988) Comprehensive functional assessment for elderly patients. *Annals of Internal Medicine*, **109**(1), 70–72.

American Nurses' Association Division on Community Health Nursing Practice (1975) *Continuity of Care and Discharge Planning Programs in Institutions and Community Agencies.* American Nurses' Association, Kansas City, Missouri.

Andrews, K. (1986) Relevance of readmission of elderly patients discharged from a geriatric unit. *Journal of the American Geriatrics Society*, **34**, 5–11.

Applegate, W.B., Akins, D., Vander Zwaag, R. *et al.* (1983) A geriatric rehabilitation and assessment unit in a community hospital. *Journal of the American Geriatrics Society*, **31**, 206–10.

Arenth, L. & Mamon, J. (1985) Determining patient needs after discharge. *Nursing Management*, **16**(9), 20–24.

Barker, W.H. (1986) Hospital-based geriatric services in Great Britain: implications for the United States. *PAHO Bulletin*, **20**(1), 1–23.

Barker, W.H., Williams, T.F., Zimmer, J.G. *et al.* (1985) Geriatric consultation teams in acute hospitals: impact on back-up of elderly patients. *Journal of the American Geriatrics Society*, **33**, 422–8.

Berkman, B. & Abrams, R.D. (1986) Factors related to hospital readmission of elderly cardiac patients. *Social Work*, **31**, 99–103.

Berkman, B., Campion, E.W. Swagerty, E. *et al.* (1983) Geriatric consultation team: alternate approach to social work discharge planning. *Journal of Gerontological Society Work*, **5**(3), 77–87.

Berkman, B., Dumas, S. Gastfriend, J. *et al.* (1987) Predicting hospital readmission of elderly cardiac patients. *Health and Social Work*, **12**, 221–8.

Berkman, B., Bedell, D., Parker, E. *et al.* (1988) Preadmission screening: an efficacy study. *Social Work in Health Care*, **13**(3), 35–50.

Blaylock, A. & Cason, C.L. (1992) Discharge planning: predicting patients' needs. *Journal of Gerontological Nursing*, **18**(7), 5–10.

Borok, G., Reuben, D., Zendle, L. *et al.* (1994) Rationale and design of a multi-center randomized trial of comprehensive geriatric assessment consultation for hospitalized patients in an HMO. *Journal of the American Geriatrics Society*, **42**, 536–44.

Bristow, O., Stickney, C. & Thompson, S. (1976) *Discharge Planning for Continuity of Care.* Publication no. 21-1604. National League of Nursing, New York.

Buck, M. & Mills, A. (1988) Time to go home. *Nursing Times*, **84**(41), 42–3.

Bull, M.J. (1988) Influence of diagnosis-related groups on discharge planning, professional practice, and patient care. *Journal of Professional Nursing*, **4**, 415–21.

Cable, E.P. & Mayers, S.P. (1983) Discharge planning effect on length of hospital stay. *Archives of Physical Medicine and Rehabilitation*, **64**, 57–60.

Campion, E.W., Jette, A. & Berkman, B. (1983) An interdisciplinary geriatric consultation service: a controlled trial. *Journal of the American Geriatrics Society*, **31**, 792–6.

Caradoc-Davies, T.H., Dixon, G.S. & Campbell, A.J. (1989) Benefit from admission to a geriatric assessment and rehabilitation unit: discrepancy between health professional and client perception of improvement. *Journal of the American Geriatrics Society*, **37**, 25–8.

Cedar, L., Thorngren, K.G. & Wallden, B. (1980) Prognostic indicators and early home rehabilitation in elderly patients with hip fractures. *Clinical Orthopaedics and Related Research*, **1**(152), 173–84.

Challis, D., Darton, R., Johnson, L. *et al.* (1991) An evaluation of an alternative to long-stay hospital care for frail elderly patients: 11. Costs and effectiveness. *Age and Ageing*, **20**, 245–54.

Congdon, J.G. (1994) Managing the incongruities: the hospital discharge experience for elderly patients, their families, and nurses. *Applied Nursing Research*, **7**, 125–31.

Corkery, E. (1989) Discharge planning and home health care: what every staff nurse should know. *Orthopaedic Nursing*, **8**(6), 18–27.

Coulton, C.J., Dunkle, R.E., Goode, R.A. *et al.* (1982) Discharge planning and decision making. *Health and Social Work*, **7**, 253–61.

Cunningham, L.S. (1984) Early assessment for discharge planning: adopting a high-risk screening program. *QRB*, **10**, 561–5.

Dacher, J.E. (1989) Rehabilitation and the geriatric patient. *Nursing Clinics of North America*, **24**, 225–37.

Davis, J.W., Shapiro, M.F. & Kane, R.L. (1984) Level of care and complications among geriatric patients discharged from the medical service of a teaching hospital. *Journal of the American Geriatrics Society*, **32**, 427–30.

Drew, L., Biordi, D. & Gillies, D.A. (1988) How discharge planners view their patients. *Nursing Management*, **19**(4), 66–70.

Dubler, N.N. (1988) Improving the discharge planning process: distinguishing between coercion and choice. *The Gerontologist*, **28**(suppl.), 76–81.

Dugan, J. & Mosel, L. (1992) Patients in acute care settings. Which health care services are provided? *Journal of Gerontological Nursing*, **18**(7), 31–7.

Ebrahim, S., Barer, D. & Nouri, F. (1987) An audit of follow-up services for stroke patients after discharge from hospital. *International Disability Studies*, **9**, 103–5.

Edwards, R.C. (1978) Professionals in 'alliance' achieve more effective discharge planning. *Hospitals*, **52**(11), 71–2.

Farren, E.A. (1991) Effects of early discharge planning on length of hospital stay. *Nursing Economics*, **9**(1), 25–30, 63.

Feather, J. & Nichols, L.O. (1985) Hospital discharge planning for continuity of care: the national perspective. In *Discharge Planning for Continuity of Care* (Eds E.G. Hartigan & D.J. Brown), pp. 71–7, 85. National League of Nursing, New York.

Felsenthal, G., Glomske, N. & Jones, D. (1986) Medication education program in an inpatient geriatric rehabilitation unit. *Archives of Physical and Medical Rehabilitation*, **67**, 27–9.

Fink, A., Siu, A., Brook, R. *et al.* (1987) Assuring the quality of health care for older persons. *Journal of the American Medical Association*, **258**, 1905–8.

Gayton, D., Wood-Dauphinee, S., de Lorimer, M. *et al.* (1987) Trial of a geriatric consultation team in an acute care hospital. *Journal of the American Geriatrics Society*, **35**, 726–36.

George, L.K. & Gwyther, L.P. (1986) Caregiver well being: a multidimensional examination of family caregivers of demented adults. *The Gerontologist*, **26**, 253–9.

Graham, H. & Livesley, B. (1983) Can readmissions to a geriatric medical unit be prevented? *Lancet*, **i**(8321), 404–6.

Haddock, K.D. (1991) Characteristics of effective discharge planning programs for the frail elderly. *Journal of Gerontological Nursing*, **17**(7), 10–14.

Hawe, P., Gebski, V. & Andrews, G. (1986) Elderly patients after they leave hospital. *Medical Journal of Australia*, **145**, 251–4.

Heller, B.R., Bausell, R.B. & Ninos, M. (1984) Nurses' perceptions of rehabilitation potential of institutionalized aged. *Journal of Gerontological Nursing*, **10**(7), 22–5, 27.

Hogan, D.B. (1990) Impact of geriatric consultation services for elderly patients admitted to acute care hospitals. *Canadian Journal on Aging*, **9**(1), 35–44.

Hogan, D.B., Fox, R.A., Badley, B.W.D. *et al.* (1987) Effect of a geriatric consultation service on management of patients in an acute care hospital. *Canadian Medical Association Journal*, **136**, 713–17.

Hunt, T.E. (1980) Practical considerations in the rehabilitation of the aged. *Journal of the American Geriatrics Society*, **28**, 59–64.

Jackson, M.F. (1984) Geriatric rehabilitation on an acute-care medical unit. *Journal of Advanced Nursing*, **9**, 441–8.

Jackson, M.F. (1989) Geriatric versus general medical wards: comparison of patients' behaviours following discharge from an acute care hospital. *Journal of Advanced Nursing*, **14**, 906–14.

Jackson, M.F. (1990) Use of community support services by elderly patients discharged from general medical and geriatric medical wards. *Journal of Advanced Nursing*, **15**, 167–75.

Jacobs, L., Fontana, R. & Albert, D. (1985) Is that geriatric patient really ready to go home? *RN*, **48**(11), 40–43.

Johnson, J. (1989) Where's discharge planning on your list? *Geriatric Nursing*, **10**(3), 148–9.

Johnson, N. & Fethke, C. (1985) Post-discharge outcomes and care planning for the hospitalized elderly. In *Continuity of Care: Advancing the Concept of Discharge Planning* (Ed. E. McClelland), pp. 229–240. Grune and Stratton, New York.

Jowett, S. & Armitage, S. (1988) Hospital and community liaison links in nursing: the role of the liaison nurse. *Journal of Advanced Nursing*, **13**, 579–87.

Kane, R.A. (1987) Assessing social function in the elderly. *Clinics in Geriatric Medicine*, **3**, 87–98.

Kane, R.L., Matthias, R. & Sampson, S. (1983) The risk of placement in a nursing home after acute hospitalization. *Medical Care*, **21**, 1055–61.

Kennedy, L., Neidlinger, S. & Scroggins, K. (1987) Effective comprehensive discharge planning for hospitalized elderly. *Gerontologist*, **27**, 577–80.

Lichtenstein, H. & Winograd, C.H. (1984) Geriatric consultation: a functional approach. *Journal of the American Geriatrics Society*, **32**, 356–61.

MacDonald, B. (1981) Geriatric rehabilitation: a change of plans. *Nursing Mirror*, **153**(13), 24–6.

MacGuire, J., Preston, J. & Pinches, D. (1987) Geriatric rehabilitation: a change of plans. *Nursing Mirror*, **153**(13), 24–6.

MacMillan, M.S. (1994) Hospital staff's perceptions of risk associated with the discharge of elderly people from acute hospital care. *Journal of Advanced Nursing*, **19**, 249–56.

McKeehan, K.M. (ed.) (1981) *Continuing Care. A Multidisciplinary Approach to Discharge Planning.* C.V. Mosby, St Louis.

McKeehan, K.M. & Coulton, C.J. (1985) A systems approach to program development for continuity of care in hospitals. In *Continuity of Care: Advancing the Concept of Discharge Planning* (Eds K. McClelland, K. Kelly & K. Buckwalter). Grune & Stratton, Orlando, Florida.

Marchette, L. & Holloman, F. (1986) Length of stay: significant variables. *Journal of Nursing Administration*, **16**(3), 12–19.

Markey, B.T. & Igou, J.F. (1987) Medication discharge planning for the elderly. *Patient Education and Counselling*, **9**, 241–9.

Meeds, B. & Pryor, G.A. (1990) Early home rehabilitation for the elderly patient with hip fracture: the Peterborough hip fracture scheme. *Physiotherapy*, **76**, 75–7.

Morishita, L., Sui, A.L., Wang, R.T. *et al.* (1989) Comprehensive geriatric care in a day hospital: a demonstration of the British model in the United States. *Gerontologist*, **29**, 336–40.

Naylor, M.D. (1990) Comprehensive discharge planning for hospitalized elderly: a pilot study. *Nursing Research*, **39**, 156–61.

Neary, S. & Kitchen, E.C. (1990) Discharge planning for the elderly: implementation of a continuing care role. *Nursing Administration Quarterly*, **14**(2), 16–21.

Neidlinger, S.H., Scroggins, K. & Kennedy, L. (1987) Cost evaluation of discharge planning for hospitalized elderly: the efficacy of a clinical nurse specialist. *Nursing Economics*, **5**, 225–30.

Nolan, M.R. (1987) The future role of day hospitals for the elderly: the case for a nursing initiative. *Journal of Advanced Nursing*, **12**, 683–90.

Packard-Helie, M.T. & Lancaster, D.B. (1989) A vital link in continuity of care. *Nursing Management*, **20**(8), 32–4.

Patterson, C. (1986) Geriatric assessment in the acute care hospital. *Health Care*, **28**(8), 25–30.

Pawlson, L.G. (1988) Hospital length of stay of frail elderly patients: primary care by general internists versus geriatricians. *Journal of the American Geriatrics Society*, **36**, 202–7.

Pellegrino, R.M. & Buckley, T.F. (1987) Hospital to home: a partnership in discharge planning. *Caring*, **6**(5), 10–13.

Pleasant, R. (1991) Developing a nursing/instructor community liaison role. *Nursing Management*, **22**(9), 70–71.

Reardon, G.T., Blumenfeld, S., Weissman, A.L. *et al.* (1988) Findings and implications from preadmission screening of elderly patients waiting for elective surgery. *Social Work in Health Care*, **13**(3), 51–63.

Reichelt, P.A. & Newcomb, J. (1980) Organizational factors in discharge planning. *Journal of Nursing Administration*, **10**(12), 36–42.

Resseler, J.F. (1991) Improving elderly recall with biomodal presentation: a natural experiment of discharge planning. *The Gerontologist*, **31**(3), 364–70.

Rock, B., Goldstein, M., Hopkins, M. *et al.* (1990) Psychosocial factors as predictors of length of stay of medicare patients under the prospective payment system. *Journal of Health Care and Social Policy*, **2**(2), 1–15.

Rorden, J.W. & Taft, E. (1990) *Discharge Planning Guide for Nurses*. W.B. Saunders, Philadelphia.

Rosenblatt, D.E., Campion, E.W. & Mason, M. (1986) Rehabilitation home visits. *Journal of the American Geriatrics Society*, **34**, 441–7.

Rubenstein, L.Z., Josephson, K.R., Wieland, F.D. *et al.* (1984) Effectiveness of a geriatric evaluation unit: a randomized clinical trial. *New England Journal of Medicine*, **311**, 1664–70.

Saltz, C.C., McVey, L.J., Becker, R.M. *et al.* (1988) Impact of a geriatric consultation team on discharge placement and repeat hospitalization. *Gerontologist*, **28**, 344–9.

Schaefer, A.L., Anderson, J.E. & Simms, L.M. (1990) Are they ready? Discharge planning for older surgical patients. *Journal of Gerontological Nursing*, **16**(10), 16–19.

Schlemmer, B. (1989) The status of discharge planning in intensive care units. *Nursing Management*, **20**(7), 88A–88P.

Schmitt, M.H., Farrell, M.P. & Heinemann, G.D. (1988) Conceptual and methodological problems in studying the effects of interdisciplinary geriatric teams. *Gerontologist*, **28**, 753–64.

Schrager, J., Halman, K., Myers, D. *et al.* (1978) Impediments to the course and effectiveness of discharge planning. *Social Work in Health Care*, **4**(1), 65–79.

Shine, M.S. (1983) Discharge planning for the elderly patient in the acute care setting. *Nursing Clinics of North America*, **18**, 403–10.

Simmons, W.J. (1986) Planning for discharge with the elderly. *QRB*, **12**(2), 68–71.

Skinner, K.M. & Tennstedt, S.L. (1994) Do characteristics of informal caregivers affect the length of hospital stay for frail elders? *Journal of Aging and Health*, **6**, 255–69.

Smith, A., Slaughter, S.E. & Berg, K. (1987) Evaluation of a geriatric rehabilitation unit. *Gerontion*, **2**(3), 15–17.

Smith, P. & Andrews, J. (1983) Drug compliance not so bad, knowledge not so good: the elderly after hospital discharge. *Age and Aging*, **12**, 236–42.

Staff (1983) Discharge planning improves after care for elderly. *Hospital Progress*, **64**(1), 22–4.

Teasdale, T.A., Shuman, L., Snow, E. *et al.* (1983) A comparison of placement outcomes of geriatric cohorts receiving care in a geriatric assessment unit and on general medicine floors. *Journal of the American Geriatrics Society*, **31**, 529–34.

Thliveris, M. (1990) A hospital wide discharge planning program. *Dimensions in Health Service*, **61**(1), 38–9.

Tierney, A.J., Closs, S.J., Hunter, H.C. *et al.* (1993) Experiences of elderly patients concerning discharge from hospital. *Journal of Clinical Nursing*, **2**, 179–85.

Tierney, A. & Closs, J. (1993) Discharge planning for elderly patients. *Nursing Standard*, **7**(52), 30–33.

Trella, R. (1991) Investigation of medicare readmissions. *Nursing Management*, **22**(5), 94.

Victor, C.R. & Vetter, N.J. (1985) A one-year follow-up of patients discharged from geriatrics and general medical units in Wales. *Archives of Gerontology and Geriatrics*, **4**, 117–24.

Wachtel, T.J., Fulton, J.P. & Goldfarb, J. (1987) Early prediction of discharge disposition after hospitalization. *Gerontologist*, **27**, 98–103.

Warshaw, G.A., Moore, J.T., Friedman, S.W. *et al.* (1982) Functional disability in the hospitalized patients. *Journal of the American Medical Association*, **248**, 847.

Waters, K.R. (1987a) Discharge planning: an exploratory study of the process of discharge planning on geriatric wards. *Journal of Advanced Nursing*, **12**, 71–83.

Waters, K.R. (1987b) Outcomes of discharge from hospital for elderly people. *Journal of Advanced Nursing*, **12**, 71–83.

Weinberger, M., Smith, D.M., Katz, B.P. *et al.* (1988) The cost-effectiveness of an intensive postdischarge care. *Medical Care*, **26**, 1092–1101.

Wertheimer, D.S. & Kleinman, L.S. (1990) A model for interdisciplinary discharge planning in a university hospital. *The Gerontologist*, **30**(6), 837–40.

Williams, T.F., Zimmer, J.G., Hall, W.F. *et al.* (1987) How does the team approach to outpatient geriatric evaluation compare with traditional care: a report of a randomized controlled trial. *Journal of the American Geriatrics Society*, **35**, 1071–8.

Wisendale, S.K. (1987) Evaluating a geriatrics program in an acute-care hospital. *Gerontologist*, **27**, 440–2.

Worth, A., Tierney, A. & Lockerbie, L. (1994) Community nurses and discharge planning. *Nursing Standard*, **8**(21), 25–30.

Acknowledgements

The chapters in this book are updated papers originally published in the *Journal of Advanced Nursing*. Listed below are references to the original versions.

1 *Health promotion: the emerging frontier in nursing* by Patricia M. King: *Journal of Advanced Nursing* (1994) **20**, 209–18.
2 *Caregivers' emotional wellbeing and their capacity to learn about stroke* by Valerie Braithwaite and Anne McGown: *Journal of Advanced Nursing* (1993) **18**, 195–202.
3 *Monitoring the pressure sore problem in a teaching hospital* by Carol Dealey: *Journal of Advanced Nursing* (1994) **20**, 652–9.
4 *The characteristics and management of patients with recurrent blockage of long-term urinary catheters* by Kathryn A. Getliffe: *Journal of Advanced Nursing* (1994) **20**, 140–49.
5 *Measuring feeding difficulty in patients with dementia: developing a scale* by Roger Watson: *Journal of Advanced Nursing* (1994) **19**, 257–63.
6 *Nurses' role in informing breast cancer patients: a comparison between patients' and nurses' opinions* by Tarja Suominen, Helena Leino-Kilpi and Pekka Laippala: *Journal of Advanced Nursing* (1994) **19**, 6–11.
7 *Evaluation of the pain response by Mexican American and Anglo American women and their nurses* by Evelyn Ruiz Calvillo and Jacquelyn H. Flaskerud: *Journal of Advanced Nursing* (1993) **18**, 451–9.
8 *Does the use of an assessment tool in the accident and emergency department improve the quality of care?* by Jane Christie: *Journal of Advanced Nursing* (1993) **18**, 1758–71.
9 *Psychosocial recovery from adult liver transplantation: a literature review* by Steven P. Wainwright: *Journal of Advanced Nursing* (1994) **20**, 861–9.
10 *Intensive care: situations of ethical difficulty* by Anna Söderberg and Astrid Norberg: *Journal of Advanced Nursing* (1993) **18**, 2008–14.
11 *Spiritual aspects of nursing* by Linda A. Ross: *Journal of Advanced Nursing* (1994) **19**, 439–47.
12 *Discharge planning: issues and challenges for gerontological nursing. A critique of the literature* by Marilyn F. Jackson: *Journal of Advanced Nursing* (1994) **19**, 492–502.

Index